# Stronger with Plants

## Regain Your Health & Youthful Energy with a Plant-Based Lifestyle

Vanita Rahman, MD
Foreword by Dr. Neal Barnard

This is a general book about nutrition and health and is not a substitute for medical care, diagnosis, or treatment. Please consult with your personal physician regarding your health, medications, and medical conditions.

Published by CitrusLLC

Illustrations and photography by Lightworks-photography.com
Author's website at www.CitrusLLC.com

# Contents

# A Note to the Reader

Please work with your physician when you start a plant-based diet. After starting a plant-based diet, you may see rapid reductions in your blood sugar and blood pressure. If you are taking medications that can affect blood pressure or blood sugar levels, it is very important that you and your physician monitor these values carefully, and adjust the medications as needed.

After you transition to a plant-based diet, please be sure to take a reliable source of vitamin B12 as outlined in the chapter on vitamins and minerals.

Please consult with your physician before starting any type of exercise program to ensure that it is safe for you to exercise.

# Acknowledgments

When I was in high school, I used to dread writing. I didn't understand how to write an essay, and I avoided classes that involved much writing. I even avoided college applications that require an essay. It wasn't until freshman year of college that I learnt to write. I am very grateful for the graduate student who taught "Contemporary American Literature," and took the time to teach me an essential skill. This book would not have been possible without his encouragement and coaching.

I would like to thank Drs. Neal Barnard, Caldwell Esselsytn, T. Colin Campbell, and Dean Ornish, for all they have done to educate us about nutrition and health. Their groundbreaking research has filled a very important gap in medical education and training. I would like to thank Dr. Neal Barnard for writing the foreword to this book, and for the incredible work that he and the Physicians Committee have done to help others.

I would like to thank my friend Micheal for introducing me to the world of plant-based nutrition. His advice forever changed my life.

He has been a trusted friend since medical school, and I am very grateful for his friendship and support.

I would like to thank my friends—Basia, Candace, Mark, and Matt —for taking the time to read my manuscript, and giving me very helpful feedback. I would like to thank Matt, who not only edited my manuscript, but whose love for reading and writing inspired me to write this book.

I would like to thank my husband and children for embarking on this plant-based journey with me. I would like to thank my husband for being an equal partner in the kitchen, and for seeking out new gadgets to ease our cooking. I would like to thank my daughter for whipping up delicious vegan desserts for us. And I would like to thank my son for always being the first in line to try our vegan creations. Eating well is a family affair, and  I couldn't have done it without them.

# Foreword

Many people are looking for better ways to improve their health. We're exercising, trying to make healthier food choices, and getting our check-ups. Still we are not quite where we would like to be, and we could use help.

If this sounds familiar, this book is the answer you have been looking for. Written by Vanita Rahman, MD, an experienced authority in medicine and nutrition, it will bring you the knowledge you need and the practical advice to put it to work. For years, Dr. Rahman has helped people lose weight and tackle a broad range of health problems, and she will help you, too.

In our research at the Physicians Committee, we have found that when people change their diets in the right way, the health payoff is often dramatic. Excess weight falls away, cholesterol levels plummet, blood pressure comes back to where it belongs, and diabetes improves and sometimes even goes away. In a 2006 study, we found that particular power comes from a plant-based diet. Not only was it more effective than a more conventional "diabetes diet;" it was also surprisingly easy to follow—with no need for calorie counting or carb limits, and plenty of delicious foods to choose from.

We have found similar results with other health conditions: people suffering with the pain of rheumatoid arthritis or migraine often find that the answer comes not from a pill, but from a diet change. When you put the right foods to work, they act like powerful medicines—with one important difference: the "side effects" of a diet change are all ones you want! You'll have more energy, a trimmer waistline, and a longer life.

In these pages you will find clear explanations of how foods will improve your health, simple ways to put their power to work, and plenty of inspiration to keep you motivated.

Neal D. Barnard, MD, FACC
President, Physicians Committee for Responsible Medicine
Adjunct Associate Professor of Medicine, George Washington University
Washington, DC

# Introduction

**W**elcome to my book!

I am Dr. Vanita Rahman, a practicing internal medicine physician, a certified nutritionist, a certified personal trainer, and an advocate for a plant-based diet. I am also a cancer survivor, a wife, and mother of twin "Tweens."

So why have I written a book about nutrition?

The easiest way to answer that question is to share my own story with you. I was born in New Delhi, India. Growing up, my family had modest means, and our diet was comprised of whole grains, legumes, fruits, and vegetables. Sodas, juices, ice creams, and chocolates were neither widely available nor economical. Our diet was naturally healthy. My family and I didn't have access to television or video games. For fun, my sister and I played outside with our friends. I was lean and healthy without thinking about diet or exercise.

In 1983, my family and I moved to the United States, and my lifestyle took a turn for the worse. All of those foods that were cost prohibitive were now easily accessible. I quickly fell in love with soda, juice, chips, and desserts and I began consuming them on a daily basis. I also gained access to 24-hour television and video games and before long I was watching soap operas for two hours after school, and devouring my favorite junk foods at the same time. Outdoor play with my friends? Mostly a relic of my past life in India.

Within 15 months, I had undergone a transformation from "lean" to "chubby." One day, as my sister and I were heading off to the pool in our swimsuits, I looked down towards my toes and saw something I had never seen before—belly fat. I was shocked! I wondered, When and how did this happen?

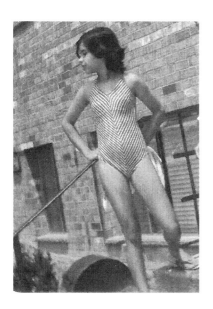 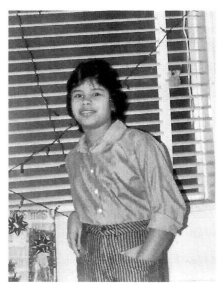

I struggled with the extra weight and belly fat for most of my adult life despite trying various exercise routines and diet plans. Each time, I would lose the weight, only to regain it within a few months.

During medical school, I started to exercise on a daily basis in order to relieve the stress of an intense academic program. I lost weight and felt great. I thought that I had discovered the key to weight loss—exercise. Unfortunately, within six months I regained all of my lost weight. However, I continued to exercise because I loved the way it made me feel.

After residency, I gave birth to my twins, and had difficulty losing the pregnancy weight. My husband and I decided to try the fabled South Beach Diet. We lost weight and thought that avoiding "carbs" was the key to maintaining a healthy weight. We were wrong. Within six months, we had regained all of our lost weight and then some. The excess weight wasn't merely a cosmetic issue—it was impacting my health. I had high blood sugar and cholesterol levels, and signs of early knee arthritis. I felt frustrated and hopeless, and chalked up the extra weight and weight-related conditions to poor genes.

A few years later, a trusted friend from medical school advised me to consider plant-based diets. My immediate reaction was to dismiss the notion. A plant-based diet seemed too extreme and didn't resonate with anything I had learned during my medical training.

Several months later, one of my patients came to see me for a lump in her neck. The lump was worrisome, and further diagnostic testing revealed that she had metastatic cancer. Sadly, my patient died a few months later. As a physician, I see many patients with many ailments, and some patients always stay in my heart. She was one of them.

A few months later, I felt a lump in my neck. I was ill with a cold at the time, and assumed that it was a reactive lymph node in response to the cold. However, the lump persisted, and I couldn't help but think of my patient. I was concerned and sought further evaluation. As I lay on the ultrasound table, I will never forget the words the radiologist said to me: "I have good news, and I have bad news. The good news is that the lump is a benign lymph node. The bad news is that you have thyroid cancer." I was terrified—I had young children and I wanted to see them grow up. Although my endocrinologist and surgeon assured me that I had an excellent prognosis, I was scared. Each time I had a scan or blood test, I was worried about recurrence. I felt helpless to control the cancer. I desperately wanted to regain control of my health.

I reconsidered my friend's suggestion to look into plant-based diets. What I learned was astounding. Researchers at some of the most prestigious institutions in the country, such as the Cleveland Clinic, Cornell University, and University of California San Francisco, had shown that plant-based diets can lead to sustainable weight loss and improvement in health. Plant-based diets have been shown to reverse diabetes, high blood pressure, and high cholesterol levels, as well as heart disease, which is the number one killer in the United States. As physicians, we stabilize heart disease temporarily, and the disease usually progresses. Reversal of heart disease virtually never happens with the traditional practice of medicine. Plant-based diets also reduce the risk of most cancers and auto-immune diseases, such as type 1 diabetes and multiple sclerosis. They are also beneficial in reducing inflammation and arthritis.

As I learned about the benefits of plant-based diets, a few questions nagged at me: Why didn't I learn about plant-based diets during my medical training and why doesn't our public health policy advocate for plant-based diets? As I explain later in the book, although the majority of deaths due to chronic disease can be prevented through lifestyle and diet changes, the majority of medical schools do not provide adequate education regarding nutrition. I will also explain why our public health policy hasn't kept pace with nutrition research.

My family and I soon adopted a plant-based diet, and the results exceeded my expectations. Within a year, my weight fell from 127 to 107 pounds, and my husband's weight fell from 180 to 155 pounds. More importantly, we have maintained the weight loss over the past few years. Our blood sugar and cholesterol levels are in the normal range. In fact, my husband's cholesterol decreased by over 80 points! He had also been suffering from obstructive sleep apnea prior to starting a plant-based diet, and his sleep apnea is now resolved. My family's allergic rhinitis and asthma are much improved. I used to suffer from three to four head colds every year—I have only had one since I switched to a plant-based diet three years ago. When I go for my scans and surveillance blood tests, I no longer feel as scared as I used to. I feel that I, rather than my genes, control my health with the diet and lifestyle choices I make.

To return to the question I posed at the start of this chapter, I wrote this book to help others do what I have done: regain control of their weight and their health.    Genes are not destiny. We can change the trajectory of our health with the lifestyle choices we make. In subsequent chapters, I will review important concepts in nutrition, medical research that supports plant-based diets, how plant-based diets compare to other popular diets such as Mediterranean and low-carb, and common concerns regarding plant-based diets.

If you find the idea of switching to a plant-based diet intimidating and overwhelming, you are not

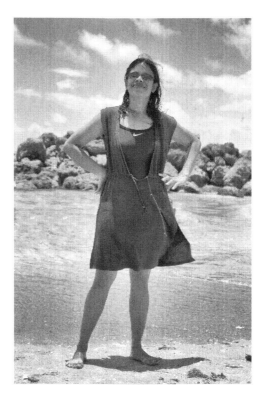

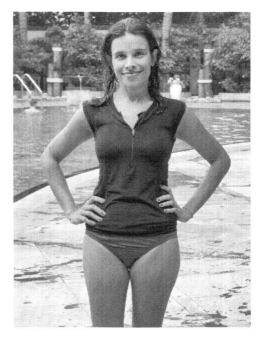

alone! I felt the same way when I first learned about it. After all, we are talking about a major lifestyle change, and the idea of making it overnight is daunting. In the book, I will provide a step-by-step guide to making a gradual transition to a plant-based diet. If you follow my advice, you too can attain and maintain a healthy weight and improve your health, without gimmicks or fads. If you don't think that you can ever fully change to a plant-based diet, then it is worth noting that the more you move towards plant-based eating, the better results you will see in your long-term weight and health goals.

*I have no financial interests to declare nor do I sell any supplements or weight-loss products.*

# Chapter 1
# What Is a Healthy Weight and Why Does It matter?

From ages 22 through 42, I exercised daily. I enjoyed jogging, step aerobics, and swimming. My friends and family told me how healthy I was because I exercised regularly. Yet my blood sugar and cholesterol levels were high, and my right knee ached if I jogged too much. My orthopedic surgeon told me that my knee was fine, but as I look back at the MRI report, I had signs of early arthritis. At the time, I thought I was taking good care of myself and was at a healthy weight. Now that I am 20 pounds lighter, I can't imagine how those extra pounds must have felt. As I compare my pictures from then to now, I can see clearly that I was heavy. Yet at the time, I felt my weight was fine because that was all I knew. How do we know whether our weight is healthy or not—is our appearance a good indicator?

## Sobering Statistics

For the past four decades, the obesity rate has been steadily rising.[1] It is now a national and global epidemic. The rise in obesity is directly linked to our deteriorating diets and more sedentary lifestyles. The following numbers shed some light on the severity of the situation:[1,2]

- Approximately 71% of American adults are overweight, and 38% of American adults are obese.
- In the U.S., 20% of adolescents between the ages of 12-19 are obese.
- Approximately 18% of American children between the ages of 6-11 are obese.
- Approximately 8% of American children between the ages of 2-5 are obese.
- Since 1980, worldwide obesity has more than doubled.
- Worldwide, 39% of adults are overweight and 13% are obese.
- Most of the world's population lives in countries where being overweight or obese causes more death than being underweight.

Being overweight or obese are much more than a matter of appearance; they are also key contributors to a number of debilitating diseases. One such disease is diabetes, which is usually caused by a combination of excess body weight, poor eating habits, and sedentary lifestyle. It not only increases one's blood sugar levels but can also lead to blindness, kidney failure, amputation of legs and feet, nerve damage, heart disease, and stroke. According to the Centers for Disease Control and Prevention (CDC), the prevalence of diabetes in the U.S. is rapidly rising among adults:[3]

- 29.1 million Americans have diabetes, that is 1 out of 11 Americans. One out of four Americans with diabetes do not know that they have the disease.

- 86 million adults have pre-diabetes. Nine out of ten pre-diabetics do not know that they have the disease.
- Without adequate weight loss, nutrition and exercise, 15-30% of pre-diabetics will develop diabetes within the next five years.
- Diabetes and its related complications accounted for $245 billion in total medical costs and lost work and wages in 2012.
- Currently, one out of three Americans will eventually develop diabetes.
- The mortality rate is 50% higher in people with diabetes.

Obesity, hypertension, diabetes, and heart disease are tightly intertwined as the same risk factors (excess weight, poor diet, and lack of exercise) lead to all four conditions. Not surprisingly then, the statistics regarding heart disease are just as alarming:

- Heart disease is leading cause of death in the U.S. for both men and women.[4]
- Over 735,000 Americans have a heart attack every year.[4]
- Every year, about 610,000 Americans die of heart disease, that is one out of every four deaths.[4]
- By the time you finish reading this page, someone will have had a heart attack in the U.S., as one occurs every every 43 seconds.[5]
- Heart disease and strokes cost America $312 billion annually in health care expenses.[5]
- 1.2 million stents are placed in the U.S. every year with a mortality of 1%.[6]
- 500,000 coronary bypass surgeries are done every year in the U.S. with a mortality rate of 1-5%.[6]

## Table 1-1 Obesity-related diseases

| Organ system | Complications[7] |
| --- | --- |
| Nervous system (Brain, spinal cord, nerves) | Stroke, dementia |
| Cardiovascular system (Heart, blood vessels) | High blood pressure, heart attacks, heart failure, poor circulation, atrial fibrillation |
| Skin | Stretch marks, hirsutism in women |
| Gastrointestinal system (esophagus, stomach, intestines, liver, pancreas) | Heartburn, fatty liver, gallstones |
| Kidneys | Kidney stones, chronic kidney disease |
| Endocrine system (hormones) | Type 2 diabetes, elevated cholesterol levels |
| Reproductive system | Polycystic ovarian system, erectile dysfunction |
| Respiratory system | Obstructive sleep apnea |
| Cancers | Endometrial, gallbladder, kidney, liver, colon, cervical, thyroid, ovarian, postmenopausal breast, leukemia |
| Musculoskeletal | Gout, osteoarthritis |
| Urinary Tract | Urinary incontinence |
| Psychosocial | Public disapproval, poverty, single status, lower education, depression |

## Health Consequences of Overweight and Obesity

As the above statistics highlight, being overweight or obese aren't merely cosmetic problems. Excess body weight wreaks havoc on virtually every organ system in our bodies. Table 1-1 outlines some of the most common diseases associated with excess body weight.

Every organ system is affected by excess weight as seen in Table 1-1. In order to fully appreciate how being overweight or obese harms our bodies, it is important to understand what the words "overweight" and "obese" mean, as well as other commonly used terms, such as Body Mass Index (BMI), abdominal obesity, and visceral fat.

## Fat Distribution and Body Types

When I speak about excess body weight, what I am really referring to is excess body fat. Think of our bodies as an enclosed space with many different types of tissues such as muscles, bones, blood, organs, skin, and fatty (aka adipose) tissue. In simplistic terms, our body weight is basically the summation of two types of weights: adipose and lean. Lean body weight is comprised of all of our body parts (bones, organs, muscles, skin, blood) except adipose tissue. Adipose tissue refers to all of the fat deposits in our bodies. It is excessive adipose tissue that leads to health problems, not excessive lean tissue.

There are two types of adipose tissues in our bodies: subcutaneous fat and visceral fat. Subcutaneous fat refers to fat deposits just under the skin and accounts for 80% of the fat in men and 90% of the fat in women.[8] Visceral fat is the fat deposited around abdominal organs, and it increases the risk of heart disease, high blood pressure, diabetes, and high cholesterol.[9] Persons with excess visceral fat are said to have abdominal, visceral, android or male pattern obesity.

When excess body fat is present, it is generally distributed in one of two patterns, and depending upon the pattern, individuals are either characterized as "apple" or "pear" shaped.[10] An apple is wider on top and narrower on the bottom. Similarly, apple-shaped persons carry most of their excess fat in their upper body, such as chest and abdomen, and hence are more likely to have abdominal obesity. Pears are narrower on top and wider on the bottom. Pear-shaped persons carry most of their excess weight in their lower body such as hips and legs. Our genes determine whether we are pear or apple shaped. While we cannot change our genes or body shape, it is imperative that we try to maintain a healthy weight and lifestyle in order to minimize the complications from excessive body fat.

> **What is your body type?** When you gain weight, do your pants feel tighter around the waist or hips? If you answer waist, then you are apple shaped. If you answer hips, then you are pear shaped.

Most men and Asian women tend to be apple shaped, while most Caucasian women tend to be pear shaped. So what is the significance of the different body shapes? While excessive body fat increases the risk for chronic diseases with both body types, the risk is particularly greater for apple shaped persons due to their greater propensity for abdominal fat.

It is important to appreciate that we cannot control where our body deposits excess fat or where it loses the fat from. When we gain or lose weight, our body stores and sheds the extra fat in a certain sequence. For example, when apple-shaped persons gain weight, the excess fat is deposited in the chest and abdomen first and later in the lower body. Similarly, when apple-shaped people lose weight, the chest and abdomen will be the last places from which they lose the excess fat. Conversely, if you are pear shaped, you will gain weight on your hips and thighs first, and lose weight from these places last. Therefore, the common adage, "a moment on the lips, a lifetime on the hips," only applies to pear-shaped persons. People often believe that they can flatten their abdomen by doing extra crunches, or slim their thighs by doing extra thigh exercises. This is simply not true. Extra abdominal or thigh exercises will further strengthen and develop the muscles in these areas. However, doing so will not reduce the surrounding fat. The only way to lose the extra fat is to eat well, exercise, and reach your ideal body weight.

## Body Mass Index (BMI)

If the real problem is excess body fat, then how do we estimate the amount of excess body fat and whether it is abdominal or subcutaneous? Computed tomography (CT) and magnetic resonance imaging (MRI) are the most accurate tools.[8] However, they are rarely used in clinical practice due to expense, as well as radiation exposure with CT and patient inconvenience with MRI. Many health clubs and personal trainers routinely use other tools to measure body fat, such as skin fold testing or impedance measurement. However, these tools do not give accurate measurements of total body fat, nor do they discriminate between subcutaneous or abdominal fat.

Rather than using expensive and inconvenient tests with potential radiation exposure, it is more cost effective to use a combination of anthropometric measurements to assess the degree and type of excess body fat. Anthropometric measurements consist of a patient's height, weight, BMI, and waist circumference. BMI is calculated and classified as follows:[9]

$$BMI = \text{Body weight (kg)} / \text{Body height (m)}^2$$

Table 1-2 outlines the BMI categories for Caucasians, Blacks, and Hispanics, and Table 1-3 outlines the BMI categories for Asians. Table 1-4 shows how waist circumference is classified based upon race.

## Table 1-2 BMI Caucasians, Blacks, & Hispanics

| Category[9] | BMI |
| --- | --- |
| Underweight | <18.5 |
| Normal | 18.5-24.9 |
| Overweight | 25 - 29.9 |
| Obese Class I | 30 - 34.9 |
| Obese Class II | 35 - 39.9 |
| Extreme Obesity | 40+ |

## Table 1-3 BMI Classification for Asians

| Category[9] | BMI |
| --- | --- |
| Overweight | 23-24.9 |
| Obese | 25+ |

## Table 1-4 Criteria for elevated waist circumference

| | Non-Asians[9] | Asians [9] |
| --- | --- | --- |
| Women | Waist circumference >= 35 inches (88 cm) | Waist circumference > 31.5 inches (80 cm) |
| Men | Waist circumference >= 40 inches (102 cm) | Waist circumference > 35.4 inches (90 cm) |

As shown in Table 1-3, Asians are classified as being overweight or obese at lower BMIs than other races. Additionally, Asian waist circumference are considered elevated at lower measurements than those of other races. The reason is that Asians have more overall body fat and abdominal fat than a Caucasian or Black person.[9] Put another way, if an Asian person and Caucasian person have the same height, weight and therefore BMI, the Asian person will have more overall fat and abdominal fat than the Caucasian person. Since it is the amount of body fat, especially abdominal fat, which increases our risk for heart disease, diabetes, hypertension and elevated cholesterol, Asians need to maintain a lower BMI than other races. Similarly, for any given waist circumference, Asians are more likely to have abdominal obesity than a person from another racial group.

While BMI is an extremely useful tool, not all BMIs are equal. Simply measuring BMI without considering other confounding variables can lead to erroneous conclusions. When interpreting BMIs, it is important to bear in mind the following caveats:

- Race matters. Asians have a greater propensity for overall body and abdominal fat then other racial groups. Hence it is advisable for Asians to maintain a lower BMI.

- Body shape and abdominal obesity matter. Apple-shaped individuals have more abdominal obesity than pear-shaped individuals. Hence, apple-shaped persons are at higher risk for weight-related complications and need to maintain a lower BMI.

- Lifestyle matters. To illustrate this principle, let's compare an elite athlete and a sedentary person with the same height, weight and therefore BMI. The elite athlete has very little adipose tissue and a higher percentage of lean body mass due to muscle development, and is therefore not at risk for weight-related conditions. The sedentary individual has a greater percentage of the body weight from excessive fat and is therefore at higher risk for weight-related complications.

- Look for evidence of lifestyle-related disease. What do I mean by this? When assessing a person's weight, it is important to evaluate if he or she already shows evidence of weight-related complications. For example, if Mr. Jones is a 40 year old Caucasian male with a BMI of 24.5 and his fasting blood sugar is 102 (normal fasting blood sugar is less than 100) and his blood pressure is 150/95 (normal < 140/90), then he already has evidence of weight-related diseases. Even though his BMI is technically in the "normal" range, lowering his BMI may reverse the elevated blood sugar and blood pressure.

# Chapter 2

# Overview of the Health Benefits of a Plant-Based Diet

**I** lived in India until age 12, where vegetables, lentils, and fruits were our staple food. My mother cooked a wide variety of vegetables on a daily basis such as okra, cauliflower, eggplant, and squash, and served them with home-made bread and rice. We had legumes on a daily basis. We occasionally had cheese and yoghurt. My favorite fruit was mango—my grandfather used to buy a large crate of mangoes and parcel them out to all of the children. After I finished my share, I would stare at my cousins while they ate theirs, hoping they would share with me. While I liked some of the vegetables and legumes, I longed for cakes, chocolates, ice cream, and soda. Growing up in a middle-income family in India in the 70's and early 80's, these items were expensive and often reserved as treats to be enjoyed on special occasions. Whenever my grandfather was invited to a wedding, my cousins and I would vie to go with him so that we could drink soda and have ice cream. After moving to the U.S. at age 12, I could enjoy chocolate, ice cream, soda, and cakes on a daily basis because they were affordable. These food items tasted great and I indulged myself. Whether in India or the U.S., I grew up eating the food that was around me without thinking about the impact it had on my health. Looking back now, I can see how fortunate I was to have been exposed to vegetables, fruits, and legumes as a regular part of my diet during my childhood.

## What Is a Whole-Food, Plant-Based Diet? What Is the Difference Between a Whole-Food Plant-Based Diet and a Vegan Diet?

A whole-food, plant-based diet is comprised of minimally processed plant-based foods such as whole grains, vegetables, fruits, legumes, nuts and seeds with minimally added fats or sugars. Such a diet has been proven to have tremendous health benefits and the focus of the diet is to eat well in order to optimize one's health.

Vegans pursue a lifestyle where all animal products are avoided for moral or ethical reasons. The emphasis in vegan eating is not necessarily on avoiding processed foods, added sugars or fats as it is in a whole-food, plant-based diet.

## What Are the Health Benefits of a Whole-Food, Plant-Based Diet?

Most chronic western diseases are diseases of lifestyle and nutrition. Current medical treatment for most chronic diseases manages the diseases without addressing the underlying causation, which is diet and lifestyle. As a result, the disease continues to progress. There is substantial research showing that a whole-food, plant-based diet can prevent and even reverse most chronic diseases. Additionally, a whole-food, plant-based diet can be delicious, satisfying and easy to follow, with the correct knowledge and tools. In the following section, I briefly summarize the benefits of plant-based eating. (Detailed information about research studies focused on plant-based eating appears in the next chapter.) Here are some of the benefits of a whole-food, plant-based diet:

- Lose weight and maintain a healthy weight.

  Research has shown repeatedly that vegetarians and vegans maintain a healthier weight than non-vegetarians.[1,2] Plant-based foods increase our metabolism, thereby increasing the number of calories we burn at rest.[1,2,3] Additionally, plant-based food are less calorically dense than animal-based foods. Ounce for ounce, plant-based foods offer more nutrients such as fiber, and fewer calories, fat and cholesterol than animal-based foods.[4]

| Chick peas 82g<br>kcal 134<br>kcal from fat 18<br>kcal from protein 29<br>Cholesterol 0<br>Fiber 6.2g | vs. | Lean steak 85g<br>kcal 170<br>kcal from fat 76<br>kcal from protein 92<br>Cholesterol 50mg<br>Fiber 0 |
| --- | --- | --- |

- Minimize and even reverse diabetes.

  Insulin is a hormone produced by pancreatic cells. It drives glucose from the blood into various body cells. When there is insufficient insulin, or if the body's cells are resistant to insulin, blood glucose level rises. Diabetes is usually diagnosed by measuring a fasting blood glucose level when a patient has not had anything to eat or drink, except water, for at least eight hours.[5]

### Table 2-1 Classification of fasting blood glucose

| Fasting blood glucose level (mg/dL) | Classification |
| --- | --- |
| < 100 | Normal |
| 100 - 125 | Pre-diabetes |
| 126 or greater | Diabetes |

Another test that is commonly used to diagnose and monitor diabetes is hemoglobin A1C (A1C). Some of the sugar in blood binds with hemoglobin, which is a protein found in red blood cells. As blood sugar levels rise, the percentage of hemoglobin bound to sugar increases. A1C represents blood sugar values over the past 8 to 12 weeks. Table 2-2 shows how A1c is used to diagnose diabetes.[5] For patients diagnosed with diabetes, an A1C is checked every three months to assess diabetic control. The goal for most diabetic patients is to maintain A1C values below seven.

### Table 2-2 Using A1C to diagnose diabetes

| Hemoglobin A1C | Classification |
| --- | --- |
| < 5.7 | Normal |
| 5.7 - 6.4 | Pre-diabetes |
| 6.5 or greater | Diabetes |

There are two types of diabetes: type 1 and type 2. Type 1 diabetes occurs in genetically-susceptible persons when the immune system gradually destroys the pancreatic cells that produce insulin. However, the risk for type 1 diabetes is not entirely genetic and environmental factors play a strong role. If type 1 diabetes was entirely genetic, we would expect a concordance rate of 100% in identical twins. (Concordance rate is the likelihood of an identical twin having the same disease.) However, when an identical twin is diagnosed with type 1 diabetes, the other twin has a 30% chance of being diagnosed within 10 years and 65% chance of being diagnosed within 20 years.[6] Hence, more than genes are playing a role.

The incidence of type 1 diabetes increases as populations move further away from the equator.[2,6] Research has shown that early exposure to cow's milk may be associated with the production of antibodies that destroy the insulin-producing cells.[2,7,8] Dairy consumption also increases as one moves further from the equator.[2] It is very likely that increased dairy consumption further from the equator accounts for the geographic variation seen in type 1 diabetes.

As individuals move from a low prevalence location to a high prevalence area, their risk of type 1 diabetes increases.[2,6] The overall incidence of type 1 diabetes is increasing in the U.S. and globally. A study from the city of Philadelphia showed that the prevalence in children less than age five increased by 70% from 1985 to 2004.[6] All of these factors point to a strong environmental cause as genes don't change with geographical relocation or in such short periods of time. Approximately 5% of diabetics in the U.S. have type 1 diabetes, which is usually diagnosed in childhood.[9] Patients with type 1 diabetes need lifelong insulin since their pancreases will not produce any.

Type 2 diabetes is lifestyle related, and accounts for 95% of cases of diabetes in the U.S. Excess body weight, poor diet and sedentary lifestyle lead to a combination of decreased insulin production by the pancreas and increased resistance to insulin. Normally seen only in adults over age 40, type 2 diabetes is now increasingly seen in children, adolescents and young adults as the prevalence of obesity grows in our youth. From 2001 to 2009, the incidence of type 2 diabetes increased by 31% in youth 10-19 years old.[10]

Patients with type 2 diabetes are traditionally treated with oral medications or insulin. There is increasing research showing that type 2 diabetes can be minimized and even reversed with a whole-food, plant-based diet.[2]  In a randomized control trial, patients with type 2 diabetes were either assigned a low-fat vegan diet, or a diet following the guidelines of the American Diabetes Association (ADA).[11] After 22 weeks, A1C measurements decreased in both groups, but the decrease was significantly greater in the vegan group. A1C decreased from 8.07 to 6.84 in the low-fat vegan group. In contrast, it decreased from 7.88 to 7.5 in the ADA group.

A Korean research study of type 2 diabetics published online in *PLoS ONE* showed similar results.[12] Korean researchers randomized patients with type 2 diabetes into two groups and followed them for 12 weeks. The experimental group followed a vegan diet and the control group followed the Korean Diabetes Association diet. A1C levels decreased from 7.5 to 6.6 in patients that were highly compliant with a vegan diet, versus 7.4 to 7.2 in the control group. It is noteworthy that medications were not changed in either group and that the vegan group was not required to restrict calories or portion size.

Researchers at Harvard followed over 200,000 participants to evaluate how a healthy plant-based diet can lower the risk of developing type 2 diabetes. Participants who ate a greater quantity of healthy plant-based foods, reduced their risk of type 2 diabetes by 34%.[13]

- Lower cholesterol.

    **Cholesterol is only found in animal-based foods. It is not found in plant-based foods**. As I will discuss further in the chapter on fats, cholesterol is essential and humans produce enough to meet their daily needs. We do not need to consume cholesterol in our foods. Dietary cholesterol raises our cholesterol levels, and excessive cholesterol levels increase our risk for cardiovascular disease. Most animal-based foods are naturally high in fat and cholesterol, while most plant-based foods are naturally low in fat and devoid of cholesterol. The combination of high levels of fat and cholesterol in animal-based foods increases blood cholesterol levels. In the China-Cornell-Oxford Project (aka The China Study), researchers compared the cholesterol levels of rural Chinese who ate a mostly plant-based diet to that of Americans whose diet is rich in animal-based foods. The average blood cholesterol was 127 mg/dL in rural Chinese who ate a mostly plant-based diet compared to a cholesterol of 217 mg/dL for the average American.[2] Many Chinese persons had blood cholesterol levels far lower than 150 mg/dL, numbers which are hardly ever seen in western populations.[2] Additionally, as detailed in the next chapter, research has shown dramatic lowering in cholesterol levels with the adoption of plant-based diets.

- Lower blood pressure.

    Plant-based diets lower blood pressure in several ways. Blood pressure is inversely correlated with the amount of dietary potassium we consume.[14] Diets low in potassium increase blood pressure while diets high in potassium reduce blood pressure. Fruits and vegetables are naturally rich in potassium, thereby increasing potassium intake and lowering blood pressure.[14] Additionally, patients who follow a whole-food, plant-based diet tend to have healthier weights, which also reduce the risk of high blood pressure.

- Minimize and reverse cardiovascular disease.

  As you will see later in Chapter 4, research has shown dramatic reduction and even reversal of coronary artery disease in patients with advanced heart disease who follow a whole-food, plant-based diet.

- Lower the risk of most cancers including breast, colorectal, and prostate.

  Breast, colorectal and prostate cancers are some of the most common cancers in the U.S. According to the World Health Organization (WHO), diet is responsible for 30% of cancers in developed countries and 20% of cancers in developing countries.[15] While there is significant media attention focused on the genetic basis for breast cancer, genetic mutations only account for 5-6% of all breast cancer cases in the U.S.[16] Hence most breast cancer cases are due to environmental factors. There is substantial research showing the connection between the consumption of animal-based foods and breast cancer. It is well established that the risk of breast cancer is proportional to the duration and level of estrogen exposure as increased estrogen exposure leads to increased risk of breast cancer. The China Study found the following correlations regarding animal food intake and breast cancer risk:[2]

  - Countries with the highest rates of animal fat intake have the highest rates of breast cancer.

- In contrast, plant fats do not affect the incidence of breast cancer.
- Higher consumption of animal foods leads to an earlier age of menarche, later age at menopause, and increased levels of estrogen during reproductive years. Animal foods are high in fat content, which is thought to increase the levels of estrogen.
- Women and young girls in rural China consume lower amounts of animal-based foods than women in western countries.
- Consequently, most girls in rural China start menstruating at 15-19 years of age, with an average age of 17 years. In contrast, the U.S. average is 11 years!
- Western women reach menopause 3-4 years later than the women in rural China.
- During reproductive years, estrogen levels in Chinese women were only about half those of western women.
- It is no surprise then that breast cancer rates in rural China are one-fifth of those seen in Western women.
- Furthermore, as women in rural China increased their intake of animal foods, the incidence of breast cancer increased.

Other researchers have shown that Bovine Leukemia Virus found in dairy milk has been linked to breast cancer.[16] Although women are often concerned that soy-based products may increase their risk of breast cancer, the opposite is true. Phytoestrogens are naturally occurring plant substances and their structure is similar to the estrogen found in our bodies. However, phytoestrogens seem to reduce the risk of breast cancer. Soy products are rich in isoflavones, a type of phytoestrogen. Asian women who consume more that 20 mg/day of isoflavones reduced their risk of breast cancer by 29%.[15] Harvard's Nurses' Health Study II, which tracked the dietary habits of 88,804 women for 10 years, showed that a diet high in animal fat increased the risk for breast cancer by 18% among all women and 21% among postmenopausal women.[18]

Similar to breast cancer, countries with the highest rates of animal food consumption have the highest rates of colorectal cancer.[2] Research has shown that plant-based foods reduce the risk of colorectal cancer, while consumption of meats increases the risk.[2] There are several reasons for this. Fiber, found only in plant-based foods, reduces the risk of colorectal cancers. Animal-based foods do not contain fiber. Meats (including red meat, chicken and fish) contain several known carcinogens, such as heterocyclic amines (HCA) and polycyclic aromatic hydrocarbons (PAH,) which are formed during the processing or cooking of meat. [15] Animal-based foods also have high levels of fat. In response to fatty meals, the gall bladder produces bile acids, which travel to the intestines in order to help with fat absorption. However, bacteria in the intestines convert these bile acids into secondary bile acids, which are carcinogenic.[15] Furthermore, animal foods promote the growth of intestinal bacteria, which convert bile acids to secondary bile acids.[15]

Most recently, the International Agency for Research on Cancer (IARC), the cancer agency of the WHO, issued a report regarding the carcinogenicity of red and processed meat. IARC defined red meat as muscle meat from any mammal such as beef, veal, pork, lamb, mutton, horse, and goat.[19] Processed meat was defined as any meat that is transformed through salting, curing, fermentation, smoking, or other processes that improve flavor or preservation.[19] Most processed meats are made from pork or beef, but may also be made from other red meats, poultry, offal, or meat by-products such as blood.[19] More than half of the meat Americans eat is red meat, and nearly a quarter of it is processed.[20]

The IARC working group consisted of 22 experts from ten countries.[21] They reviewed more than 800 studies regarding the association between meat intake and 12 dozen different cancers, in various countries and in populations with diverse diets.[21] The IARC concluded the following regarding processed meat[19,21]:

- Processed meat is a human carcinogen.
- For every 50 grams of daily consumption of processed meat, the risk of colorectal cancer increases by 18%. What comprises 50 grams of processed meat?
    - 6 bacon strips
    - 2 ham slices
    - 1 hot dog
    - 5 slices of hard salami
    - Eating any of these servings on a daily basis will increase the risk of colorectal cancer by 18%.
- Processed meat consumption was also associated with stomach cancer.
- Worldwide, about 34,000 cancer deaths per year are due to diets high in processed meat.

IARC reached the following conclusions regarding red meat[19,21]:

- Red meat is probably carcinogenic to humans.
- The association between red meat and cancer is strongest for colorectal cancer, but was also seen for pancreatic and prostate cancer.
- For every 100 grams of daily consumption of red meat, the risk of colorectal cancer increases by 17%.

- Worldwide, about 50,000 cancer deaths per year may be due to diets high in red meat.

Prostate cancer is also associated with higher levels of animal food intake. As with breast cancer, high fat content in animal foods increases testosterone levels, which in turn increases the risk for prostate cancer. Phytoestrogens, high in soy products and legumes, have been shown to reduce the risk for prostate cancer.[22] A growing body of research is showing that dairy products increase the risk of prostate cancer. In the Harvard Physicians' Health Study, which followed 20,885 men for 11 years, two and one-half servings of dairy products each day increased the risk of prostate cancer by 34%, compared to men who had less than one-half of a serving daily.[23]

- Reduce the risk of autoimmune diseases such as type I diabetes and multiple sclerosis.

In autoimmune diseases, the body's immune system gradually attacks and destroys the body's cells, most likely due to a combination of genetic and environmental factors. Common examples of such diseases include type 1 diabetes, multiple sclerosis, thyroiditis, and vitiligo. Multiple sclerosis (MS) is a devastating disease in which the immune system gradually damages the nervous system and leads to severe disability, such as an inability to walk or see. Currently, there is no cure, and available treatment options are complex and less than optimal.

Much research has been done into the disease, and many of the patterns observed with type 1 diabetes are also seen with MS. Incidence of MS increases with distance from the equator, and with greater consumption of cow's milk.[2] The disease isn't entirely due to genetic factors, since the concordance rate in identical twins varies from 20-39%.[24] Dr. Roy Swank, who served as the head of the Division of Neurology of the University of Oregon Medical School (Oregon Health & Science University) for 22 years, hypothesized that the geographic variation in MS was due to changes in diet rather than sun exposure or the electromagnetic fields of the earth. He followed 144 MS patients for 34 years, and recommended that they consume less than 20 g/day of saturated fat. Of the sub-group of patients who began the diet earlier in the course of their disease, about 95% remained mildly disabled for the next thirty years and only 5% died. But 80% of the patients with early-stage MS who did not adhere to the diet died of MS.[2]

Given the link between the level of saturated fat consumption and the impact on MS, it is noteworthy that plant-based diets are naturally low in saturated fats (and animal-based diets are high in them).

- Reduce the risk of osteoporosis.

Most of us have grown up believing that we should drink as much dairy milk as possible, since it is supposed to be good for us and our bones. However, this message has largely been promoted by the dairy industry, which targets young children along with their parents and teachers.[2] The dairy industry provides "educational material" to schools such as posters, websites and activities that promote dairy consumption and the benefit of dairy products.[15] The problem is that science does not support the health benefits of milk and other dairy products.

Consider the example of osteoporosis, which is a disease of the bones usually seen in older adults. In osteoporosis, bone architecture changes, and bones become brittle and prone to fracturing. Such osteoporotic fractures usually occur in the hip, spine, or wrist. Bone mineral density has been used as a surrogate to estimate the degree of osteoporosis, and to estimate the risk for fracture. As bone density decreases, the risk of fracture increases.

The traditional thinking has been that inadequate calcium intake increases the risk for osteoporosis. For years, women and older adults have been advised to increase their intake of calcium through diet or supplements to minimize their risk of osteoporosis and fractures. However, research has shown that the countries with the highest incidence of cow's milk consumption have the highest incidence of hip fractures.[2] Research has also shown that as the ratio of animal protein to plant protein increases, the incidence of hip fractures increases.[2] While calcium supplements are over-the-counter drugs, they are not benign, as they increase the risk for kidney stones, heart disease, constipation, and gastrointestinal discomfort.[25] Calcium supplements also interfere with the absorption other medications, such as thyroid hormone and iron.[25] Most recently, two studies published in the *British Medical Journal* in October 2015 shed more light on this topic. A systemic review of the literature showed that calcium intake via the diet or supplements did NOT reduce the incidence of osteoporotic fractures.[26] Another systemic review and meta-analysis of the literature showed that dietary and supplemental calcium increased bone mineral density by only about 0.6-1.8% after one year, and no further increases were seen thereafter.[27] Such an increase in bone density is minimal and highly unlikely to impact risk of fracture.[28]

As I have outlined in this chapter, there is tremendous evidence associating animal-based foods with increased risk of cancer, osteoporosis, auto-immune disease, heart disease, high blood pressure, diabetes, elevated cholesterol levels, and excess body weight.

On the other hand, significant research shows that the risk of all of these diseases is reduced by consuming a whole-food, plant-based diet. At this point, it may seem tempting to decipher which nutrients in plants reduce disease risk or which chemicals in animal foods increase disease risk, and then manipulate the putative agents in our foods. However, it is important to appreciate that plant-based foods contain many hundreds of nutrients that are beneficial to us, many of which we have yet to identify. Similarly, animal foods likely contain hundreds of chemicals that are harmful to us, many of which are yet unidentified. It is the composite healthfulness of plant-based foods that are beneficial to our health, rather than any one ingredient.[2] Similarly, the overall composition of animal foods increases inflammation and oxidative stress in our bodies, thereby leading to innumerable chronic diseases.[2]

# Chapter 3
# Prominent Research Studies Supporting Whole-Food, Plant-Based Diets

In this chapter, I summarize the most notable studies supporting whole-food, plant-based diets. Notwithstanding the fact that these studies were conducted at some of the most prestigious medical institutions in the United States, and their results were published in highly-acclaimed medical journals, I didn't learn about them during my medical training, and most of my fellow physicians don't know about them.

As I review research findings, it will be helpful to review some commonly used medical terms:

- **Coronary arteries**: arteries that supply blood to the heart.
- **Coronary artery disease**: Over time, blockage develops in the coronary arteries. This blockage may not cause any symptoms, or may cause chest pain with gradual, partial

blockage or a heart attack with sudden and complete blockage.

- **Angina**: chest pain caused by partial blockage in coronary arteries.
- **Myocardial Infarction** (aka heart attack): caused by sudden, complete blockage in one of the coronary arteries.
- **Angioplasty**: A cardiologist inserts a catheter through the groin and into the heart. The catheter then opens the blockage in the coronary artery. A stent is sometimes inserted afterwards to keep the artery open.
- **Coronary artery bypass surgery**: A very complex open heart surgery where one or more of the blocked coronary arteries is replaced with an artery from elsewhere in the body.
- **Cardiovascular disease**: includes coronary artery disease, stroke, peripheral vascular disease.
- **Peripheral vascular disease**: caused by blockage in arteries which supply blood to the legs. When the blockage is gradual, pain occurs in the legs with exertion. This is known as **claudication**. When the blockage is sudden and complete, all   blood flow stops and the affected area may need amputation.
- **Deep vein thrombosis (DVT)**: a clot forms in the veins which carry blood from the legs to the heart. The clot prevents blood from leaving the leg properly, thereby leading to a red, swollen and painful leg.
- DVT is different from claudication. In claudication, there is an obstruction of blood flow in the arteries which carry blood from the heart to the leg. Whereas in DVT, the obstruction is in veins which carry blood from the leg to the heart.
- **Stroke**: caused when blood flow to certain parts of the brain stops abruptly.

# Turning Cancer on and off with Nutrition in Laboratory Animals[1]

Dr. T Colin Campbell is Jacob Gould Schulman Professor Emeritus of Nutritional Biochemistry at Cornell University. He has shown how nutrition can turn cancer on and off in laboratory animals even when they are infected with potent carcinogens.

- Aflatoxin and Hepatitis B Virus (HBV) are known carcinogens that cause liver cancer.
- Rats infected with aflatoxin develop cancer if the protein source is casein (dairy milk protein), but they not if the protein source is gluten.
- Furthermore, for rats fed solely with casein, as casein concentration increases from 5% to 20%, cancer increases. In contrast, as the dietary casein content decreases from 20% to 5%, cancer decreases.
- Mice infected with HBV develop liver cancer if they are fed casein but not gluten.

# China-Cornell-Oxford Project (aka The China Study)[1]

"The China Study" is the largest and most comprehensive study of human nutrition. The project was a collaboration between Cornell University, Oxford University and the Chinese Academy of Sciences. In the early 1970's, as the premier of China was dying of terminal cancer, he commissioned a nationwide survey of cancer. Over 650,000 workers surveyed 880 million Chinese citizens. The survey led to the production of an atlas that showed the incidence of over four dozen diseases, including various cancers, as well as cardiovascular and infectious diseases. One of the study's most noteworthy findings was that cancer incidence in China varied by as much 100 fold among different regions. (By comparison, the prevalence of cancers in different regions in the U.S. only varies by 2 or 3 fold.) The regional variation was quite a surprise since 87% of Chinese population are of the same ethnic group, the Han group. Therefore the variation in cancer incidence was not due to genetic factors but environmental or lifestyle factors.

In 1983, Cornell University, Oxford University and Chinese Ministry of Health initiated "The China Study" to understand the connection between lifestyle and environmental factors, and the regional variation in cancer incidence noted in China in the early 1970's. Researchers studied 6,500 Chinese persons in 100 rural to semi-rural Chinese counties. Rural locations were chosen since the lifestyle and diet had not changed in these counties since the early 1970's when the disease atlas was established. Additionally, 90-94% of adults remained in the same counties since early 1970's. Hence the diet and lifestyle of Chinese living in these rural counties from 1983 could be correlated with the incidence of cancer and chronic diseases in the early 1970's.

"The China Study" showed the following dietary patterns for the average Chinese as compared to the average American with the same body weight:

- Americans ate 1989 kcal/day whereas Chinese ate 2641 kcal/day.
- Americans got 34-38% of their daily kcal from fat, whereas Chinese got 14.5% of daily kcal from fat.
- American daily fiber consumption was 12 g/day, whereas for Chinese it was 33 g/day.
- Americans ate 91g of protein daily, whereas Chinese ate 64g of protein daily.
- Americans consumed 10-11% of their daily calories from animal proteins, whereas the Chinese consumption was 0.8%.
- Average American animal protein intake was 70 g/day and 7.1 g/day for average Chinese.

- American daily ingestion of iron was 18 mg/day whereas it was 34 mg/day for Chinese.

The study showed the following correlations between diet and diseases:

- Average Chinese blood cholesterol was 127 mg/dL, whereas average American cholesterol was 217 mg/dL.
- As Chinese people ate a more westernized diet (higher in animal foods, lower in plant-based foods), their total cholesterol and LDL (bad) cholesterol increased.
- As cholesterol levels increased, not only did the incidence of cardiovascular disease increase, so did the incidence of most cancers.
- As total cholesterol increased from 90 mg/dL to 170 mg/dL, the incidence of the cancers of the liver, rectum, colon, lung, breast, childhood leukemia, brain, stomach and esophagus increased.
- Coronary heart disease mortality was seventeen times higher among American men than rural Chinese men.
- Breast cancer-related mortality was five times higher in America than in rural China.
- Increased animal food intake was associated with earlier age at menarche (age 15-19 in China vs. age 11 in U.S.), more estrogen exposure during reproductive years, and later age at menopause. All of these factors results in increased lifetime estrogen exposure and increased incidence of breast cancer.
- Reduced fiber (found only in plant-based foods) intake and increased animal food intake was associated with increased incidence of bowel diseases, such as constipation and colon cancer.
- Regions with lower fruit intake had cancer rates that were five to eight times higher.

- HBV infection rates are very high in rural China: 12-13% vs 0.2-0.3% in the U.S. Chronic HBV infection can cause liver cancer, and liver cancer rates were higher in rural Chinese who consumed a diet high in animal-based foods.

As the Chinese diet changed from a traditional plant-based diet to a more western animal-based diet, the population's blood cholesterol, incidence of heart disease, and cancer increased.

## The Lifestyle Heart Trial

Dr. Dean Ornish and his colleagues at the University of California San Francisco School of Medicine conducted a randomized, controlled clinical trial from 1986-1992 in patients with preexisting coronary artery disease. Through lifestyle intervention, they were able to reduce the frequency, duration and severity of chest pain. Even more impressively, they reduce the amount of blockage in the coronary arteries. The results of the study were published in *The Lancet*, a very well respected medical journal, in 1990. Briefly, the study showed the following:[2]

- Forty-eight patients were enrolled in the clinical trial, and all of them had coronary artery disease documented by a coronary angiogram.
- Twenty-eight patients were assigned to the lifestyle intervention group and they were prescribed a low-fat vegetarian diet, tobacco cessation, moderate physical exercise, stress reduction techniques, and a support group. The prescribed diet was comprised of fruits, vegetables, legumes, soybean products and grains without caloric restriction. No animal-based foods were allowed except for egg whites and one serving of nonfat milk or yogurt daily. Approximately 10% of the calories came from fat, 15-20%

of the calories came from protein and 70-75% of the calories came from complex carbohydrates. Cholesterol intake was limited to less than 5mg/day. Notably, none of the patients in either group were taking cholesterol-lowering medications.

- Twenty patients were assigned to the control group and were not prescribed lifestyle changes but were free to make them.
- Patients were followed for one year, and at the end of the year, the following results were noted in the lifestyle intervention group:

  - Without the use of cholesterol lowering medications, total cholesterol decreased by 24.3%. In contrast, total cholesterol decreased by 5.3% in the control group
  - LDL cholesterol decreased by 37.4%, compared to a reduction of 5.9% in the control group.
  - Frequency of chest pain decreased by 91%. In contrast, chest pain frequency increased by 165% in the control group.
  - Duration of chest pain decreased by 42% but it increased by 95% in the control group.
  - Chest pain severity decreased by 28% and it increased by 39% in the control group.
  - The average blockage in coronary arteries in the lifestyle intervention group decreased by 4.5% but increased in the control group by 5.4%.

Due to the impressive reductions in cholesterol and regression in coronary artery disease, the study was extended for another four years. The results of this trial were published in the *Journal of the American Medical Association (JAMA)* in 1998. At the end of the additional four-year study period (5 years total), the following results were noted:[3]

- Patients in the lifestyle intervention group had lost an average of 12.8 pounds whereas the control group had no weight change.
- In both groups, the average LDL cholesterol decreased by 20%. However, none of the patients in the lifestyle intervention group were taking cholesterol-lowering medications; in the control group, 60% of the patients were taking such medications.
- The average blockage in coronary arteries in the lifestyle intervention group decreased by 7.9% but increased in the control group by 27.7%.
- The 7.9% decrease in coronary artery blockage translated into significant reductions in the number of cardiac events. Cardiac events are defined as any of the following: heart attack, angioplasty, bypass surgery, heart related hospitalization or heart related death.
- In the lifestyle treatment group, there were 0.89 cardiac events per patient. Whereas, in the control group, there were 2.25 cardiac events per patient.

The most notable finding in The Lifestyle Heart Study is that the patients in the lifestyle intervention group lowered their cholesterol, blockage in coronary arteries and cardiac events **without** taking any cholesterol lowering drugs. In contrast, patients in the control group followed standard medical care, and despite 60% of the them taking cholesterol-lowering medications, their coronary blockage and cardiac events increased. It is important to note that cholesterol-lowering medications are not benign medications. They can lead to liver damage, muscle damage, and in extreme cases, kidney failure.

## Dr. Caldwell Esselstyn and the Cleveland Clinic

Dr. Caldwell Esselstyn, Jr., is a prominent surgeon at the Cleveland Clinic where he has served as the president of the staff, member of the Board of Governors, chairman of the Breast Cancer Task Force and head of Section of Thyroid and Parathyroid Surgery.[1] His other accolades include a gold medal in the 1956 Olympics for rowing, and Bronze Star as an Army surgeon in the Vietnam War.[1] Disillusioned with the standard treatment in the U.S. for cancer and heart disease, and intrigued by research showing the role nutrition played in chronic disease, he conducted his own research study at the Cleveland Clinic.[4]

- Between 1985-1988, 24 patients enrolled in the trial. All patients had known coronary artery disease.
- All patients started a whole-food, plant-based diet and took minimal amounts of cholesterol-lowering medications. All animal-based foods and oils were prohibited except for skim milk and nonfat yogurt. Fat intake was restricted to less than 10%.
- Six patients dropped out of the study within the first 12-18 months. By 1998, these non-adherent patients suffered a total of 13 new cardiac events.
- Eighteen patients continued the study.
  - Twelve years into the study, none of the adherent patients experienced any progression of coronary disease or new cardiac events.
  - Five years into the study, 11 of the 18 patients had coronary angiograms that showed the disease was arrested in all and regressed in eight of the patients. Prior to the study, all 11 of these patients had severe progressive coronary artery disease and were receiving state-of-the-art care at the Cleveland Clinic.

- During the eight years prior to starting the study, these 11 patients had suffered collectively a total of 37 cardiovascular events as follows:
  - Fifteen cases of increased angina
  - Six cases of angiographically determined disease progression
  - Six cases of coronary artery bypass surgery
  - Four myocardial infarctions
  - Three strokes
  - Two angioplasty procedures
  - One abnormal (worsening) stress test.
- Average cholesterol decreased from 246 mg/dL to 145 mg/dL.
- Of the nine patients who suffered from chest pain prior to the study, the chest pain resolved in two patients and decreased in seven.
- In the 12 years following the initiation of the study, only one person discontinued the diet.

Impressed by the study results, a physician colleague approached Dr. Esselstyn for treatment in 1996. He was a 44-year-old surgeon in otherwise good health who had suffered a heart attack. An angiogram showed that the blockage in his coronary artery was not amenable to treatment by angioplasty or bypass surgery. He started Dr. Esselstyn's plant-based dietary program without any cholesterol-lowering medications. Thirty two months later, his blood cholesterol had decreased from 159 mg/dL to 89 mg/dL and the blockage in his coronary artery was completely reversed.[5]

Encouraged by the results of the initial small study, Dr. Esselstyn conducted a larger study that showed similar improvement in cardiovascular disease with a plant-based diet:[6]

- 198 patients with known cardiovascular disease self-enrolled in the study after learning about Dr. Esselstyn's work through their physicians, word of mouth, or prior research findings.

- All were prescribed a plant-based diet comprised of fruits, legumes, vegetable, whole grains and free of meat, fowl, dairy, seafood, processed oils, avocados or nuts, sugary foods, excess salt.
- Average follow-up was 44 months.
- 89% of the patients adhered to the diet.
- Of the 198 patients, 21 patients that did not adhere to the diet had the following outcomes:
  - Eleven had further cardiovascular events: two strokes, four angioplasties, one heart transplant, three bypass surgeries, one surgery for peripheral vascular disease.
  - Two patients died from heart-related reasons.
  - Eight patients remained stable.
  - None of the patients improved.
- Of the 198 patients, 177 patients adhered to the diet with the following outcomes:
  - Average weight loss was 18.7 pounds.
  - Improvement was noted in 144 patients.
    - Angina resolved in 104 of 112 patients.
    - Further testing showed reversal of coronary disease in 39 patients.
    - Claudication improved in the one patient who had it prior to the study.
    - Twenty-seven patients were able to avoid angioplasty or bypass surgery that had previously been recommended.
  - Fifteen patients remained stable.
  - Eighteen patients had worse outcomes.
    - Of these, 15 were not related to nutrition or progression of cardiovascular disease.
    - Three had progression of cardiovascular disease.

- Five patients died from causes not related to heart disease or diet.

As Drs. Esselsytn and Ornish have clearly proven with their clinical research, a whole-food, plant-based diet can halt and even reverse the coronary artery disease which is the leading cause of death in the U.S. The average fee for an angioplasty procedure is $31,000, with an average mortality rate of 1%.[8] The average fee for a heart bypass surgery is $46,000, with a mortality range of 1-5%.[8] In contrast, lifestyle intervention with a whole-food, plant-based diet does not require any fad diets, medications or procedures. Furthermore, there is no known morbidity or mortality associated with following a whole-food, plant-based diet. Indeed, there is no other medication or surgical procedure that delivers such huge health benefits and cost savings, and without any risk to the patient.

## Research Study of Adventist Church Members

Researchers at Loma Linda University studied the diet of Adventist church members and correlated it with BMI and type 2 diabetes risk.[9] An advantage of a research study in the Adventist population is that the rates of tobacco use are extremely low (1.8%) in this group, and tobacco in known to impact BMI and diabetes risk. From 2002-2006, the diets of 60,903 Adventist church members in the U.S. and Canada were analyzed. As shown in Table 3-1, as the diet changed from vegan to non-vegetarian, the average BMI and prevalence of type 2 diabetes increased. The increased risk of type 2 diabetes with higher amounts of animal-based food intake persisted, even after adjusting for other confounding factors such as physical activity, sleep, education, and income.

## Table 3-1 Study of Adventist church members

| Diet | Definition | BMI | Prevalence of type 2 diabetes (%) |
|------|-----------|-----|-----------------------------------|
| Vegan | Dairy, seafood, poultry, meat eaten less than once per month | 23.6 | 2.9 |
| Lacto-ovo vegetarian | Dairy and /or eggs eaten at least once a month<br><br>Seafood, poultry, meat eaten less than once per month | 25.7 | 3.2 |
| Pesco-Vegetarian | Dairy, eggs and fish eaten at least once a month<br><br>Poultry, meat eaten less than once per month | 26.3 | 4.8 |
| Semi-vegetarian | Dairy, eggs, meat eaten at least once a month but less than once a week | 27.3 | 6.1 |
| Non-vegetarian | Dairy, eggs, meat eaten at least once a week | 28.8 | 7.6 |

# Chapter 4

# Impact of Eating Animal-Based Foods on Our Environment and Fellow Animals

Americans are amongst the top consumers of animal-based foods. In 2014, the total consumption of beef, poultry, pork and lamb in the U.S. was 90 kg per capita, second only to Australia at 90.2 kg per capita.[1] In contrast, total consumption in the European Union and India were 64.8 kg and 3.3 kg per capita, respectively.[1] The consumption of animal-based foods has a tremendous negative impact on our health, and the processes used to produce these foods cause suffering of farm animals, lead to antibiotic resistance, drain valuable resources, damage our environment, and contribute to climate change.

Industrial food animal production (IFAP) produces almost all of the meat, dairy products and eggs in the U.S.[2] Under IFAP operations, thousands of cattle, pigs, and chickens are confined to a single facility where they have very limited space and mobility.[2] Due to the highly unsanitary living conditions, animals are at high risk for infection and are given continuous low doses of antibiotics to prevent infection and bolster growth. These antibiotics make their way from animal manure into the ground water system, and eventually into people. The sheer volume of antibiotics being used leads to antibiotic resistance in bacteria that are potential human pathogens. According to the Johns Hopkins University's Center for a Livable Future, 80% of the antibiotics sold in 2009 were used for livestock and poultry, and 20% were used for humans.[3]

Raising livestock drains valuable resources as it requires a large amount of land, water, feed, and fertilizer. According to research data:

- About 30% of the total ice-free surface of the earth's land is used to raise chickens, pigs, and cattle for human consumption.[4]
- According to the Environmental Working Group (EWG), 167 million pounds of pesticides, 17 billions pounds of nitrogen fertilizer, and 149 million acres of cropland are needed to produce livestock feed in the U.S. annually.[5]
- About 1,600 - 2,500 gallons of water are needed to produce one pound of feedlot beef.[2]
- According to David Pimental of Cornell University's College of Agriculture and Life Sciences, seven billion livestock in the U.S. consume five times as much grain as is consumed by the entire U.S. population.[6]
- All of the grain currently fed to U.S. livestock could feed nearly 800 million people.[6]
- Cattle ranching has been linked to four-fifths of the deforestation across the Amazon rainforest.[6]

Production and consumption of all foods generate greenhouse emissions. However, the emissions for animal-based foods are significantly higher. Full lifecycle emissions represent all of the greenhouse gases emitted during the production, processing, transportation, consumption, and disposal of a food item. EWG measures full lifecycle emissions for various foods and expresses them as a ratio:[5]

Emissions for food X =
kilogram of carbon dioxide equivalents emitted (kg CO2e)/
kilogram of food X consumed (kg)

According to EWG, lamb, beef and cheese have the highest lifecycle emissions ratios at 39.2, 27.0, and 13.5 kilos of CO2e per kilo consumed, respectively.[5] In contrast, tomatoes and lentils have the lowest lifecycle emissions ratios at 1.1 and 0.9 kilos of CO2e per kilo consumed, respectively.[5] In a 2006 report, the United Nations' Food and Agriculture Organization estimated that the livestock industry was responsible for about 18% of the greenhouse gases generated by humans.[4]

In addition to contributing to greenhouse gases, livestock waste leads to environmental pollution. According to the Environmental Protection Agency (EPA), American livestock generated 500 million tons of manure in 2007, which is three times the amount of waste generated by the entire U.S. population.[5] While manure can be a valuable nutrient for plants, excess manure overwhelms the sewage systems and leads to contamination of groundwater, rivers, streams, and the oceans.[5] According to the EPA, animal waste from confined feeding operations has contaminated more than 34,000 miles of rivers and 216,000 acres of lakes and reservoirs in the U.S.[5] As animal waste decomposes, it releases dust, smog odors, and toxic gases, all of which damage the air quality and jeopardize the health of local workers and residents.

Despite the dire consequences to our health, farm animals, and the environment, human meat consumption continues to increase. From 1971 to 2010, the size of the population grew by 81%, while meat production tripled to 600 billion pounds.[7] Global meat production is expected to double by the year 2050 to about 1.2 trillion pounds annually.[7]

# Chapter 5
# What about Other Diets Such as Mediterranean, Low-Carb, Paleo, and Okinawan?

There has been considerable interest amongst the media and public about the Mediterranean, Okinawan, and low-carbohydrate diets. These diets are popular because people perceive them to be more compatible with their current way of eating. Generally, they restrict one or two food groups, which can seem more manageable. In this chapter, I will explore the science and efficacy of these popular diets. As I mentioned before, in my quest for the correct diet, I myself have tried a low-carbohydrate diet only to realize that I could not sustain it long term, and that I was not getting the benefit that I expected from it.

## Mediterranean Diet

When evaluating a Mediterranean diet, we should examine the following aspects:

- What constitutes a Mediterranean diet?
- How effective is a Mediterranean diet?
- Since the Mediterranean diet was first labeled as a heart-healthy diet, how has it changed in the subsequent decades?
- How have these dietary changes impacted health?

What Is a Mediterranean Diet?

The phrase, "Mediterranean diet," doesn't refer to a specific diet, but to the dietary patterns of populations bordering the Mediterranean Sea. Seventeen countries share a border with the Mediterranean Sea, and they all have different cultures, diets, and eating habits. However, all of their varying diets do   rely mostly on plant-based foods, with smaller amounts of animal-based foods. The following studies have provided information about the composition of the traditional Mediterranean diet:

- After World War II, the Rockefeller Foundation evaluated the diet of the people of Crete, a Greek island with very low rates of coronary heart disease at the time. Closer analysis of the Cretan diet revealed that is was primarily plant-based. Only seven percent of the daily calories came from animal-based foods and the remaining from plant-based foods.[1]
- Ancel Keys is a pioneering American physiologist and researcher who established the epidemiological link between cholesterol and heart disease. Keys evaluated the diet of the people inhabiting Naples in the 1950s. His research showed that people in Naples had low levels of cholesterol and low incidence of heart disease. The notable exception were rich

people who ate meat every day rather than every week or two. In this affluent group that consumed meat frequently, cholesterol levels were higher, as was the incidence of heart disease.[2]

- The Seven Countries Study started in the 1950s and continues to collect data from the following countries: Finland, Netherlands, Italy, Greece, Japan, United States, and the former Yugoslavia. Data from the three countries that border the Mediterranean Sea (Italy, Greece, Yugoslavia) showed that the Mediterranean diet during the 1960s was primarily plant-based and included large quantities of bread, pastas, and vegetables.[1] Fruits were served as desserts. Cheese and meat were sprinkled on the foods, and modest amounts of meat or fish were consumed once or twice a week.[2] This is in stark contrast to the way most people in the U.S. and Mediterranean eat today, with significant quantities of dairy, poultry, and meat products consumed on a daily basis.[1]

- A study by the European Atomic Energy Commission from 1963 to 1965 showed that Southern Italians consumed a diet that was mostly plant-based, whereas the diet of rich and Northern Italians was similar to that of Northern Europeans and included far more animal-based foods.[1] As the consumption of meat and dairy products increased from Southern to Northern Italy, so did the incidence of heart disease.[2]

## How Effective Is the Mediterranean Diet, How Has it Changed over the Years, and How Have These Changes Impacted Health?

The traditional Mediterranean diet associated with a low incidence of coronary heart disease was primarily plant-based and included large quantities of grains, vegetables, fruits, and plant-based fats, with minimal amounts of dairy products, meat, and seafood. Over the years, the production and consumption of animal-based foods has increased significantly in Mediterranean countries, while the consumption of plant-based foods has decreased. As the Mediterranean people have changed their eating habits from a predominantly plant-based diet to a more animal-based diet, their rates of high blood pressure, high cholesterol levels, diabetes, heart disease, and diet-related cancers have increased.[1]

The following three research studies provide important information about the efficacy of a Mediterranean diet in preventing disease. The first study also gives data about how the diet has changed since it was first recognized as a healthy diet, and the impact these changes have had on health.

I. Research study investigating the changes in the Cretan diet from 1960 to 1991 and the subsequent impact on health

This research study, which was published in 1996 in the journal *Angiology*, evaluated how the health of rural Cretan men changed from 1960 to 1991 as their diet changed. Over the years, the Cretan diet has changed from a predominantly plant-based one to one encompassing more animal-based foods. In conjunction with this change, the consumption of bread, vegetables, and fruits has decreased, while the consumption of meat, fish, and cheese has increased. As the diet of the Cretan people changed, so did their risk factors for cardiovascular disease and the incidence of cardiovascular disease. These changes are shown in Table 5-1.[3]

## Table 5-1 Changes in the health of rural Cretan men from 1960 – 1991

| | 1960 | 1991 | Notes |
|---|---|---|---|
| % of population with systolic blood pressure > 140 | 42.6% | 45.2% | 29% of Americans have high blood pressure |
| % of population with diastolic blood pressure > 90 | 14.9% | 33.1% | |
| Mean total cholesterol | 203 mg/dL | 226 mg/dL | Average cholesterol in the China Study was 126 mg/dL |
| % of population with total cholesterol > 260 mg/dL | 12.8% | 28.6% | 14% of Americans have total cholesterol > 240 mg/dL |
| % of population with coronary artery disease | 0.7% | 9.5% | |
| % of population with major cardiovascular disease | 8.8% | 19.1% | |

When healthcare providers measure blood pressure, they record two numbers: systolic and diastolic. Systolic blood pressure refers to the upper number in the blood pressure measurement, and a value above 140 is considered elevated. Diastolic blood pressure refers to the lower number in the blood pressure measurement, and a value above 90 is considered elevated. As shown in Table 5-1, a significant number of Cretan men had elevated systolic and diastolic blood pressures in 1960, 42.6% and 14.9%, respectively. As the diet changed from 1960 to 1991, the prevalence of elevated systolic blood pressure increased marginally but the prevalence of diastolic blood pressure more than doubled. To give some perspective to these numbers, 29% of American adults had high blood pressure in 2015.[4]

The mean total cholesterol in Cretan men was 203 mg/dL in 1960, and it increased to 226 mg/dL in 1991. In contrast, in the China Study, the average cholesterol was only 127 mg/dL among rural Chinese who ate a mostly plant-based diet.[5] In 1960, 12.8% of Cretan men had total cholesterol greater than 260 mg/dL, and this percentage more than doubled to 28.6% in 1991. In comparison, 14% of Americans have total cholesterol levels greater than 240 mg/dL.[6] As explained in Chapter 9, the cholesterol levels of Cretan men in 1960 and 1991 are quite high, and the only safe total cholesterol levels are those less than 150 mg/dL.

The phrase "cardiovascular disease" encompasses many diseases, including coronary heart disease, other heart diseases, stroke, and peripheral arterial disease. Although the prevalence of coronary heart disease in rural Cretan men in 1960 was only 0.7%, almost 10% had some type of major cardiovascular disease. As the dietary patterns changed from 1960 to 1991, the incidence of both coronary heart disease and cardiovascular disease increased significantly. By1991, almost 10% of Cretan men had coronary heart disease, and almost 20% had a major cardiovascular disease.

This study is notable for two reasons. First, it shows that the incidence of high blood pressure, high cholesterol levels, and cardiovascular disease was quite significant in Cretan men in 1960 when they were eating the traditional Mediterranean diet. Second, the incidence of all of these disease grew as the consumption of animal-based foods increased.

## II. The Lyon Diet Heart Study

This was a randomized controlled trial that evaluated the effectiveness of a Mediterranean diet in the secondary prevention of cardiovascular disease.[7,8] "Secondary prevention" refers to the prevention of further cardiovascular events in patients with known or pre-existing cardiovascular disease. The trial started in 1988, and approximately 600 people were enrolled. Half of the patients were prescribed a Mediterranean diet and the remaining were told to continue their usual diet (control group). The results after 46 months of the study period are shown in Table 5-2.

### Table 5-2 Results of the Lyon Diet Heart Study

|  | Mediterranean diet group | Control group |
| --- | --- | --- |
| Number of persons | 302 | 303 |
| Cardiovascular outcomes | 90 | 180 |
| % of patients who remained free of cardiovascular events | 75% | 60% |
| Blood pressure, cholesterol, blood sugar levels | No significant changes in either group | |

As shown in Table 5-2, there were no significant differences in blood pressure, cholesterol, or blood sugar levels in either group. The Mediterranean diet reduced the number of cardiovascular events by 50%. More people in the Mediterranean diet group remained free of cardiovascular events—75% vs. 60% in the control group. While these results are encouraging, it is important to note that 25% of patients consuming a Mediterranean diet continued to have further cardiovascular events.

Let's contrast these results with those of plant-based interventions. In Dr. Esselstyn's study, patients with known cardiovascular disease were prescribed a low-fat, plant-based diet and were followed for 44 months. Of the 198 participants, 177 adhered to the diet and cardiovascular disease progressed in only three of them, approximately 1.7% of the patients.[9]

Comparing the results of the Lyon Study with Dr. Esselstyn's study, a Mediterranean diet reduces the risk of recurrent cardiovascular events in patients with known cardiovascular disease. However, it isn't as effective as a low-fat, plant-based diet.

III. The Predimed Study

This study, which began in 2003, was a randomized trial to evaluate the effectiveness of a Mediterranean diet in the primary prevention of cardiovascular disease.[10] "Primary prevention" refers to the prevention of cardiovascular events in patients who do not have known cardiovascular disease. Patients were divided into three study groups:

- Mediterranean diet with increased intake of extra-virgin olive oil (EVOO Group)
- Mediterranean diet with increased intake of nuts (Nuts Group)
- Low-fat diet. Prior to the study, the low-fat group was consuming 39% of daily calories from fat. After starting the study, this percentage declined to 37%.[11]

There were approximately 2,500 persons in each group, and patients were followed for an average of 4.8 years. The study results are shown in in Table 5-3.

### Table 5-3 Results of the Predimed Study

| | Nuts group | EVOO group | Low-fat group |
|---|---|---|---|
| Rate of stroke per 1,000 person years | 3.1 | 4.1 | 5.9 |
| Heart attacks | No significant differences between the three groups | | |
| Death from cardiovascular disease | No significant differences between the three groups | | |
| Death from any cause | No significant differences between the three groups | | |

As shown in Table 5-3, neither type of Mediterranean diet reduced the rate of heart attacks, nor did it reduce the incidence of death from cardiovascular disease or any cause. Both Mediterranean diets reduced the risk of an initial stroke. The reduction was 47% in the nuts group and 30% risk reduction in the EVOO group. It is important to note that the participants in the low-fat diet group were not consuming a low-fat diet as they reduced their fat intake from 39% of total daily calories to 37%.[11] Such high levels of fat intake are not consistent with a low-fat diet.

Summary of the Mediterranean diet

The traditional Mediterranean diet was predominantly a plant-based diet. Compared to other Western populations, the risk of coronary heart disease was lower in patients consuming a traditional Mediterranean diet. However, the incidence of high blood pressure, high cholesterol levels, and major cardiovascular disease were significant. Over the past decades, the Mediterranean diet has changed significantly, with the population consuming fewer plant-based foods and a larger quantity of animal-based food. Congruent with these changes, the incidence of high blood pressure, high cholesterol levels, coronary heart disease, and cardiovascular disease have increased in the Mediterranean population.

## Okinawan Diet

Okinawa, in south-west Japan, has long been recognized as a region with some of the highest rates of longevity and centenarians. As Table 5-1 shows, the average and maximum Okinawan life spans exceed those in Japan and America.[12]

## Table 5-1 Average and maximum life spans

|  | Average life span | Maximum life span |
|---|---|---|
| **Okinawa** | 83.8 | 104.9 |
| **Japan** | 82.3 | 101.1 |
| **United States** | 78.9 | 101.3 |

Cardiovascular disease is the leading causes of death in the United States. Mortality rates from coronary artery disease are significantly lower in Okinawa compared to those of Japan and the U.S., as shown in Figure 5-1.[12] Mortality rates from various cancers are also significantly lower in Okinawa as illustrated in Figures 5-2 and 5-3.[12]

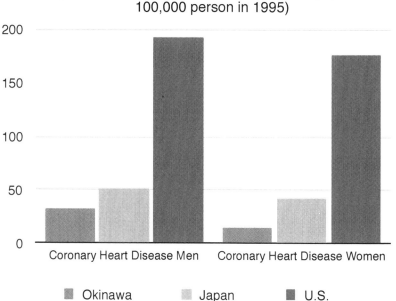

Figure 5-1 Coronary artery disease mortality (deaths/ 100,000 person in 1995)

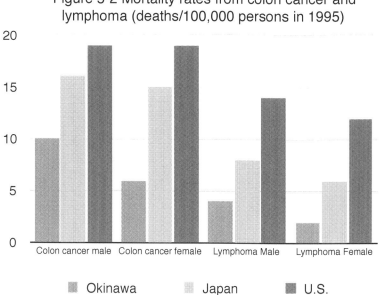

Figure 5-2 Mortality rates from colon cancer and lymphoma (deaths/100,000 persons in 1995)

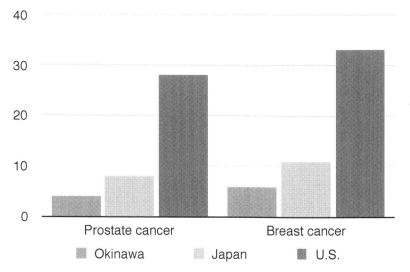

Figure 5-3 Mortality rates from prostate and breast cancers (deaths/100,000 persons in 1995)

## Table 5-2 Okinawan vs. Japanese diets

| | Okinawa 1949 | Japan 1950 |
|---|---|---|
| Total calories | 1785 | 2068 |
| Total weight in grams | 1262 | 1057 |
| Total carbohydrate in grams (% of calories) | 382 (85) | 409 (79) |
| Total protein in grams (% of calories) | 39 (9) | 68 (13) |
| Total fat in grams (% of calories) | 12 (6) | 18 (8) |
| Sweet potatoes in grams (% of calories) | 849 (69) | 66 (3) |
| Other vegetables including tomatoes and papaya (% of calories) | 116 (3) | 235 (3) |
| Fruits in grams (% of calories) | <1 (<1) | 44 (1) |
| Rice in grams (% of calories) | 154 (12) | 328 (54) |
| Other grains in grams (% of calories) | 38 (7) | 153 (24) |
| Legumes in grams (% of calories) | 71 (6) | 55 (3) |
| Sugars in grams (% of calories) | 3 (<1) | 8 (1) |
| Oils in grams (% of calories) | 3 (2) | 3 (1) |
| Nuts/seeds in grams (% of calories) | <1 (<1) | <1 (<1) |
| Fish in grams (% of calories) | 15 (1) | 62 (4) |
| Meat and poultry in grams (% of calories) | 3 (<1) | 11 (<1) |
| Eggs in grams (% of calories) | 1 (<1) | 7 (<1) |
| Dairy in grams (% of calories) | <1 (<1) | 8 (<1) |

The decreased mortality rates and increased longevity in Okinawa have been attributed to a healthy diet and active lifestyle. What is the traditional Okinawan diet and how did it differ from the one in mainland Japan? Table 5-2 compares the composition of the traditional Okinawan and Japanese diets.[12]

As seen in Table 5-2, the traditional Okinawan diet was primarily a plant-based diet, with animal based foods accounting for just 1-2% of the daily caloric intake. The diet was rich in sweet potatoes and other vegetables, rice and other grains, and legumes such as soy. There was minimal consumption of added sugars, oils, nuts, or seeds.

The mainland Japanese consumed more calories with a smaller mass of food, i.e., their diet was more calorically dense. Compared to the Okinawans, the mainland Japanese consumed a greater amount of their daily calories from rice, fish, meat, poultry, eggs, and dairy. In contrast, they consumed a lesser amount of their daily calories from sweet potatoes and legumes. These dietary changes accounted for the increased amounts of fat, protein, and caloric density of the mainland Japanese diet.

Since World War II, the Okinawan diet and lifestyle have become more westernized. The first fast-food restaurant in Japan opened in Okinawa in 1963, and Okinawa now has more fast-food restaurants per capita than the rest of the country.[13] Table 5-3 shows how the Okinawan diet has changed over the years.[14] Okinawans are now consuming more animal-based and processed foods, which translates to  more calories from fat and protein and fewer calories from healthy carbohydrates. Consumption of sodium has more than tripled, while consumption of potassium has declined by over 50%. As we will see later in the book, both of these phenomena increase blood pressure.

The westernization of the Okinawan diet has taken a tremendous toll on the health of the local population. In 1949, the average adult Okinawan BMI was a lean 21.2, which increased to 23.3 and 25 in 1972 and 1998, respectively.[12] Today, half of Okinawan men in their 40s are obese.[13] Furthermore, the Okinawan longevity is a thing of the past, and younger Okinawans now have a shorter life span than the national average. In 2005, the Okinawan life expectancy at birth was 78.64 years compared to 78.79 years nationally.[15] Thirty percent of Okinawan men die before reaching 65.[13] In 1995, Okinawa had the highest longevity of all 47 Japanese prefectures. However, its ranking fell to 26th place by the year 2000.[13]

**Table 5-3 Changes in the Okinawan diet**

|  | Traditional | Modern |
|---|---|---|
| Carbohydrates (% daily calories) | 85% | 58% |
| Protein (% daily calories) | 9% | 15% |
| Fat (% daily calories) | 6% | 27% |
| Saturated fat (% daily calories) | 2% | 7% |
| Cholesterol (mg/1000 kcal) | - | 159mg |
| Sodium | 1113 mg | 3711 mg |
| Potassium | 5199 mg | 2155 mg |

Summary of the Okinawan Diet

The traditional Okinawan diet associated with longevity and low mortality rates was primarily a plant-based diet, with only 1-2% of the daily calories coming from animal-based foods. As the diet of the Okinawan people became more westernized, the consumption of animal-based, processed, and fast-food increased, along with a subsequent decrease in health and longevity.

## Low-Carbohydrate Diets

Many popular diets, such as Atkins and South-Beach contend that carbohydrates are behind the obesity epidemic and that limiting the intake of carbohydrates, while increasing the amount of dietary fat and protein will improve health. These diets have become popular because they lead to rapid weight loss. However the weight loss is not sustainable, and it is due to a combination of a temporary reduction in calories that results from eliminating major food groups such as grains, and from the water loss due to excessive protein consumption. When people consume more protein than the body needs, the excess nitrogen found in protein is eliminated by the kidneys. In order to accomplish this, the kidneys excrete water along with the nitrogen. Thus, most of the weight loss is due to water loss. As people reintroduce grains into their diet, they tend to regain the weight.

Research has shown that low-carbohydrate diets do not improve health, and can worsen cholesterol levels, blood flow through critical arteries, and increase mortality. Pertinent study findings are outlined below:

- A research study published in the *Annals of Internal Medicine* in 2010 evaluated the impact of low-carbohydrate diets on mortality. This study also differentiated the impact of low-carbohydrate diets that were animal based from those that were plant based. Researchers followed 85,168 women in the Nurses' Health Study for 26 years, and 44,548 men in the Health Professionals Follow-up Study for 20 years. What they found was that animal-based, low-carbohydrate diets were associated with increased overall and cardiovascular mortality, whereas plant-based, low-carbohydrate diets were associated with decreased overall and cardiovascular mortality.[16]
- A meta-analysis published in 2013, reviewed all research studies that compared the mortality and incidence of cardiovascular disease in patients consuming low-carbohydrate

diets versus those who consumed high-carbohydrate diets. The analysis found that the overall mortality rate increased by 30% amongst those consuming low-carbohydrate and low-carbohydrate, high-protein diets. The analysis also indicated that such diets did not reduce the risk of cardiovascular disease and might even increase the risk long-term.[17]

- A research study published in the *British Journal of Nutrition* in 2013, evaluated the impact of low-carbohydrate, high-protein, high-fat diets on blood flow through small arteries.[18] The researchers studied 247 persons without know cardiovascular disease, who were at intermediate to high risk for developing it. Persons who consumed low-carbohydrate, high-protein, high-fat diets had poorer blood flow in small arteries. Blood flow through small arteries correlates with flow in coronary and carotid arteries that provide blood to the heart and brain, respectively, and can predict future cardiovascular events.

- A case report published in the *Journal of the American Dietetic Association* detailed the story of a healthy man who developed symptomatic cardiovascular disease and erectile dysfunction after starting the Atkins Diet.[19] The patient was a healthy 51-year-old man who was physically active and did not smoke. He had a computed tomographic scan of his coronary arteries prior to starting the diet, and it showed no evidence of heart disease. He started the Atkins Diet because his weight had increased from 63.6 kg to 67.1 kg. His cholesterol levels, weight, and clinical symptoms before and after starting the Atkins Diet are shown in Table 5-4. As shown in the table, the patient's total and LDL cholesterol levels increased after starting the Atkins diet. He also developed erectile dysfunction and chest pain after starting the diet. Erectile dysfunction shares the same risk factors as cardiovascular disease, and often precedes the development of symptomatic cardiovascular disease. A coronary angiogram was performed after he developed chest pain, and it showed blockages in several arteries. Cholesterol levels usually decrease with weight loss. Low-carbohydrate diets are the exception to this rule, as cholesterol levels increase in 30% of patients who adopt a low-carbohydrate diet.[19] The increase in total and LDL cholesterol levels is most likely due to the fact that low-carbohydrate diets are high in saturated fat and cholesterol, and low in fiber.

Table 5-4 Cholesterol levels and health status before and after starting Atkins diet

| | 6 months before starting Akins diet | Atkins diet started | 29 months on Atkins diet | 2 months after stopping Atkins diet and starting low-fat diet |
|---|---|---|---|---|
| **Weight (kg)** | 63.6 | 67.1 | 63.6 | 61.7 |
| **BMI** | 21.3 | 22.6 | 21.3 | 20.7 |
| **Total cholesterol (mg/dL)** | 146 | | 209 | 146 |
| **LDL cholesterol (mg/dL)** | 85 | | 127 | 81 |
| **HDL cholesterol (mg/dL)** | 53 | | 53 | 52 |
| **Erectile dysfunction** | No | | Yes | No |
| **Chest pain** | No | | Yes | No |
| **Cardiovascular imaging** | Normal computed tomographic coronary artery calcium score | | Coronary angiogram shows blockage in several arteries | |

Summary of Low-Carbohydrate Diets

Low-carbohydrate diets are popular amongst dieters trying to lose weight because they often lead to rapid weight loss. The weight loss is due to water loss and significant decrease in the grain intake. Dieters often regain the lost weight as they reintroduce grains into their diet. As outlined above, low-carbohydrate diets do not improve health and can worsen cholesterol levels, reduce blood flow through critical arteries, and increase mortality.

## Paleo Diet

The Paleo diet attempts to replicate the diet eaten by early human ancestors in the Paleolithic Era. The diet assumes that during the Paleolithic times, early humans ate a diet composed of wild animals and plants, and didn't consume any cultivated animal- or plant-based foods such as dairy, legumes and grains. Proponents of the Paleo diet claim that the increased prevalence of obesity and lifestyle-related diseases is due to the consumption of processed and refined foods. While there are many versions of the Paleo diet, the basic premise is to eat a diet of lean meats, fish, eggs, nuts, fruits, and vegetables, while avoiding grains, dairy, legumes, and processed sugars.

Some aspects of the Paleo diet are healthy, such as eating fruits and vegetables, and avoiding processed sugars and dairy products. However, other aspects are detrimental, such as eating meats, fish, and eggs, and avoiding grains and legumes. As we will see later in the book, whole grains and legumes are an essential part of a healthy diet.

A research study published in 2014 in the *International Journal of Exercise Science* evaluated the effects of a Paleo diet on cholesterol levels, weight, and percentage of body fat.[20] Forty four healthy adults consumed a Paleo diet for 10 weeks, while participating in a hight-intensity, CrossFit-based, exercise program. As see in Table 5-5, though the participants lost weight and body fat, their lipid profile worsened. Weight loss usually results in the lowering of blood cholesterol. What is concerning here is that the cholesterol levels increased despite weight loss and regular physical exercise. This is most likely due to the consumption of meat, eggs, and seafood, which contain high levels of cholesterol and saturated fat, and the avoidance of grains and legumes, which contain high levels of fiber that helps to eliminate cholesterol from the body. Almost any diet will lead to temporary weight loss. However, the weight loss should be sustainable and lead to improvement in health.

### Table 5-5 Effect of a paleo diet on blood cholesterol levels

|  | Before | After 10 weeks of paleo diet |
| --- | --- | --- |
| Total cholesterol | 168.8 | 178.9 |
| LDL cholesterol | 93 | 105 |
| Ratio TC/HDL | 3.0 | 3.3 |
| Percentage body fat | 24.3% | 20.7 |
| Body weight | 80.7 kg | 77.5 kg |

# Chapter 6

# Commonly Cited Barriers to Plant-Based Eating

Few years ago, a lovely new family moved into our neighborhood. Interestingly, they were following a plant-based diet due to family health history and concerns. I loved cheese, milk, and yoghurt, and didn't understand how or why anyone would give those up. The new neighbors seemed healthy, but I was skeptical of their plant-based diet—it seemed extreme. My new neighbor invited me to several dinner parties at her home where there was a wide variety of delicious plant-based food. Eating this food seemed quite enjoyable! Soon thereafter, my family embarked upon our own plant-based lifestyle. We are now good friends with our plant-based neighbors, and I am grateful for the positive influence they have had on our lives. In this chapter, I will address the concerns and questions that I had when I first learned about plant-based diets.

## How Will I Get My Protein and What About Avoiding Carbs?

No two nutrients have led to more confusion in popular dieting culture than carbohydrates and protein. As I will outline in the following chapters, healthy carbohydrates WERE NEVER the villain, and a high-protein diet is not the savior. We only need about 10% of our daily calories to come from protein, an amount which is easily met by most plant-based foods. A sensible and balanced plant-based diet can provide us with all of the essential nutrients, including protein.

## Plant-Based Diets Will Be Hard to Follow Long Term

It can seem daunting to follow a plant-based diet in today's western society, primarily because most people have grown up eating animal-based foods. Once you have learned the basic nutrition concepts, you will see that it is relatively easy to adhere to a plant-based way of eating. Most grocery stores and restaurants in the U.S. have ample plant-based foods to choose from. Additionally as Drs. Ornish, Esselstyn, and Barnard have demonstrated in their research studies, patients are willing to accept and adhere to a plant-based diet in the long-term. In Dr. Esselstyn's study of patients with severe coronary heart disease, 71% of patients adhered to a plant-based diet for over 12 years!

For those who fear that following a plant-based diet will be challenging, I say:

- Living with diabetes is tough. Taking daily shots of insulin or suffering from diabetes-related blindness, kidney failure, amputation, or nerve damage is tough.
- Suffering from chest pain or a heart attack or a stroke is tough.

- Taking multiple medications with various drug interactions and side effects is tough. I routinely see patients taking over 20 medications, which they have trouble paying for and keeping track of.
- Undergoing angioplasty or heart bypass surgery is tough.
- Watching loved ones suffer from chronic disease is tough.

## Plant-Based Diet Means Eating Boring Salads

While the stereotypical image of plant-based eating can be a cold and boring salad, nothing is further from the truth! You can look forward to eating all sorts of pastas, casseroles, stir fry, burgers, soups, tacos, burritos, pancakes, crepes, waffles, cereals, desserts, etc. With the basic nutritional information I will provide in the next four chapters, you can easily modify most recipes into a healthy whole-food, plant-based version. I have provided some of my family's favorite recipes in Chapter 11. Another great source is the website for Physicians Committee for Responsible Medicine (PCRM.org), which has many wonderful recipes.

## Plant-Based Diets Are Not for "Strong" Men

Some of the most influential men in the country follow a plant-based diet:[1,2] President Bill Clinton, CNN's Dr. Sanjay Gupta, Dr. Kim Williams (President of the American College of Cardiology), Woody Harrelson, Usher, Mike Tyson, David Carter (defensive lineman for the Oakland Raiders).

Bill Clinton has said this about a vegan diet, "changed my life. I might not be around if I hadn't become a vegan. It's great."[3]

## If Plant-Based Eating Is Better for Me, then Why Doesn't My Doctor or Government Recommend It?

Here an analogy to tobacco is helpful. While no health care provider or regulator today will argue about the dangers of tobacco use, this was not always the case. The earliest research paper linking tobacco use to cancer was published in 1930.[4] Over the ensuing years and decades, more research conclusively linked tobacco use with cancer and increased mortality. However, the first Surgeon General's report warning of the dangers of tobacco use was not issued until 1964, and cigarette boxes were not required to have warning labels until 1965.[4] Smoking was not banned on commercial flights until 1990.[5] Doctors and patients used to routinely smoke in hospitals, and smoking was not banned from hospitals until 1993.[6] It took decades for our government to issue decisive policy warning the public of the dangers of tobacco use despite mounting scientific evidence.

Unfortunately, we are facing the same situation with animal-based foods. There is tremendous scientific evidence regarding the health benefits of plant-based eating and the health hazards associated with animal-based foods. However, due to competing interests and aggressive lobbying from the beef, poultry, pork and dairy industries, there has been little change in our food policy. In response to pressure the Physicians Committee for Responsible Medicine, the U.S. Department of Agriculture (USDA) revealed in 2000 that 6 of the 11 members (including the chairman) of the U.S. Dietary Guidelines Committee had ties to the meat, dairy, or egg industry.[7] Additionally, the agricultural subsidies provided by the federal government encourage the production of animal-based foods over that of healthier fruits, vegetables, whole grains, and legumes.

Between 1995 and 2005, the USDA doled out $245 billion dollars in agricultural subsidies.[8] How did the government allocate this money?[9]

- 63% to the meat and dairy industries.
- 20% to grain production.
- 15% to sugar, starch, oil and alcohol.
- 2% to nuts and legumes.
- Less than 1% to the production of fruits and vegetables.

Further complicating the situation is that medical schools provide physicians with very little education or training in nutrition. As I mentioned in the introduction, only 27% of medical schools provide the minimum 25 hours of nutrition education recommend by the National Academy of Sciences.[10]

The fact that more physicians are not advising their patients to adopt a whole-food, plant-based diet has a simple explanation: few physicians know much about it.

# Chapter 7
# **Brief Nutrition Outline**

In this chapter, I will give a very brief overview of nutrition. In subsequent chapters, I will review each nutrient in depth.

## **Macronutrients vs. Micronutrients[1]**

We eat two basic types of nutrients: macronutrients and micronutrients. There are three types of macronutrients: carbohydrates, proteins, and fats. Macronutrients provide energy and we need to eat tens to hundreds of grams of them daily. Some macronutrients are essential while most are not. In nutrition, the word "essential" refers to nutrients that our bodies cannot make and must be ingested in our diet. In the following chapters, I will review which macronutrients are essential.

Micronutrients are comprised of vitamins and minerals. While they do not provide energy and we only need to eat a few micro or milligrams of them daily, they are essential.

## Table 7-1 Macronutrients vs. micronutrients

|  | **Macronutrients** | **Micronutrients** |
|---|---|---|
| **Subtypes** | Carbohydrates<br>Proteins<br>Fats | Vitamins<br>Minerals |
| **Provide Energy** | Yes | No |
| **Daily need** | Tens to hundreds of grams | Micro or milligrams |
| **Essential** | Some | Yes |

## Food Energy and Kcal[1]

You have presumably heard the phrase "calories" when it comes to food. What do calories really mean? A calorie is a scientific unit used to measure heat energy, much like grams or ounces are used to measure weight. How do nutrition scientists determine how much energy a food item provides? They use specialized chambers to burn the food and calculate the amount of heat it generates.

1 kilocalorie (kcal) = amount of heat needed to heat 1 kg of water by 1 degree celsius

1 kilocalorie = 1000 calories

While the scientific term for the energy related to food is kilocalorie, the phrase "calorie" is used instead on food labels and in popular culture. To clarify, when food labels say "calories," what they are really referring to is kilocalories. In this book, I will use the terms kilocalories, kcal and calories interchangeably.

For example, if an apple has 100 kcal, it means that burning the apple in a specialized chamber would heat the temperature of 100 kg of water by one degree Celsius. Different macronutrients provide different amounts of kilocalories as outlined the Table 7-2.

### Table 7-2 Energy in macronutrients

| Macronutrient | Energy (kcal/g) |
|---|---|
| Carbohydrate | 4 |
| Protein | 4 |
| Fat | 9 |
| Alcohol | 7 |

As shown in Table 7-2, fats provide more than twice as many kilocalories per gram as carbohydrates or proteins. Although alcohol is not technically a nutrient, it does provide kilocalories, and I have listed it for completeness.

# Chapter 8
# Carbohydrates - Friend or Foe?

**W**hen I speak with people about nutrition, the nutrient that causes the most confusion is the carbohydrate. Diets like South Beach, paleo, and Atkins have vilified carbohydrates and many lay persons genuinely believe that "carbs" lead to weight gain. In this chapter, I explain that carbohydrates are not one homogenous group of nutrients but a rather diverse group. Additionally, I clarify the differences between healthy and unhealthy carbohydrates. Healthy carbohydrates not only prevent weight gain, but are also essential to our health.

## Sources and Types of Carbohydrates

Carbohydrates are naturally abundant in all plant-based foods, and are found to a limited extent in dairy products. Carbohydrates are not found in poultry, red meats, or seafood. Carbohydrates are sub-divided into two groups: simple and complex.

Simple carbohydrates are called "simple" because they are small molecules that are easy for our body to digest. We ingest two simple carbohydrates in our foods: sucrose and lactose. Simple carbohydrates are also known as sugars because they are naturally sweet. Sucrose is sweeter than lactose. Sucrose is found naturally in all plant-based foods and lactose is found naturally in some dairy products. Both sucrose and lactose contain glucose, which is the basic unit of energy in our bodies. Some of the cells in our bodies, such as those in the brain, cannot work without glucose.

Complex carbohydrates are called "complex" because they are very large molecules, and it is more difficult for the body to process and digest them. We ingest two complex carbohydrates in our foods, starch and fiber, which are only found in plant-based foods.

## Table 8-1 Types of carbohydrates

|  | Carbohydrate | Source |
|---|---|---|
| Simple (aka sugars) | Sucrose | All plant-based foods |
|  | Lactose | Dairy |
| Complex | Starch | All plant-based foods |
|  | Fiber | All plant-based foods |

All plant-based foods provide a combination of simple and complex carbohydrates: sucrose, starch and fiber. Dairy products only provide the simple carbohydrate lactose. Let's now review each of these carbohydrates in more detail.

## Sucrose

As I mentioned earlier, sucrose is a simple carbohydrate or sugar, and it is sweet. Sucrose is found naturally in all plant-based foods, and the amount of sucrose in a food item determines its natural sweetness. Fruits and beets have the most sucrose and are therefore naturally sweet. Vegetables, legumes, and grains have less sucrose and are therefore less sweet. Legumes comprise all lentils and hard beans, such as chick peas, kidney beans, black beans, etc.

Table sugar is pure sucrose, and it is made by extracting sucrose from sugar cane or beets. During the production of table sugar, only sucrose is extracted and all of the other nutrients in sugar cane or beets are lost. There are many other types of sweeteners available, such as brown sugar, granulated sugar, powdered sugar, corn syrup, high fructose corn syrup, fructose, maple syrup, honey, juice concentrate, and agave. Food manufacturers use different types of sweeteners in different foods depending upon the consistency and ease of use. While the various sweeteners may have subtle differences in their chemical composition and flavor, they are all essentially similar to table sugar in terms of their effects on our bodies. No one sweetener is better or worse than another as they all provide simple sucrose without any other nutrients.[1]

Is sucrose good for us? The answer depends entirely on the quantity of sucrose, and whether sucrose is found naturally in the food or added to the it. Foods that naturally contain sucrose, such as all plant-based foods, have minimal quantities of sucrose and are full of other nutrients such as fiber, starch, protein, vitamins, and minerals. Fruits, vegetables, grains, and legumes have minimal amounts of sucrose and consumption of these foods is beneficial. While fruits are very nutritious, fruit juices should be avoided as most of the fiber and fiber-bound nutrients are lost during the juicing process. When we lose the fiber bulk during juicing, the same amount of sucrose is now concentrated in a smaller volume. Hence juices are sweeter than the original fruit, and it is very easy to consume large quantities of sucrose from fruit juices.

When we consume foods with added sugar, such as desserts or sweetened beverages, we are consuming a very large amount of sucrose without any other healthful nutrients. American consumption of added sugar has steadily increased over the years, and with that increased consumption has come the growing problem of excess body weight. For example, from 1970 to 1997, soda consumption more than doubled.[2] In 1997, the average American was drinking 54 gallons of soda per year, of which 40 gallons were non-diet, delivering 60,000 calories and 3,700 teaspoons of sugar, per person.[2] Generally speaking, approximately one pound of human body fat is equivalent to 3500 kcal, and 60,000 kcal in the form of soda translate into 17 pounds of excess fat.[3]

Desserts and sweetened beverages are obvious sources of added sugar. However, restaurants and food manufacturers often add large quantities of sugar to other foods, such as pasta sauces, cereals, salad dressings, and fruit-flavored yogurts. Cereal, which was once a healthy meal, is now often loaded with added sugar. From the late 1800s to early 1940s, cereal sold by most of the big brands was mildly sweetened.[2] However, starting in 1949, more and more sugar was added to cereal in order to increase its appeal to children. By 1956, sugar comprised more than 50% of the ingredients in many cereals.[2] Sadly, Americans have been consuming an unprecedented amount of added sugar. It is the consumption of added sugar that leads to excess weight, not the consumption of minimal amounts of sucrose that is found naturally in fruits and other plant-based foods.

## Starch

Starch is a very large and complex molecule made up of anywhere from hundreds to thousands of glucose molecules attached together. Plants store energy in the form of starch by stringing together glucose molecules. When we eat plant-based foods, our body breaks apart the bonds attaching the glucose molecules together, and all of the glucose molecules are then available for us to use for energy. Starch is found in all plant-based foods, and is most abundant in grains, which are an important source of energy for most people around the world. Is starch healthy for us? Similar to sucrose, the form in which we eat starch determines whether it is healthy for us or not. Consuming starch found in whole grains (reviewed later in chapter), legumes, fruits, and vegetables is healthy for us because these foods are also rich in other nutrients such as fiber, protein, vitamins, and minerals. Additionally, these food groups are naturally low in sucrose. On the other hand, consuming starch in refined grains (reviewed later in chapter), such as most commercially-prepared breads, white rice, or white pasta, is unhealthy because these grains are devoid of many important nutrients. Similarly, consuming starch in baked desserts is unhealthy because desserts are made with refined grains and loads of added sugars, with few if any nutrients. Over the years, most of the starch intake in the U.S. has been in the form of refined grains or baked desserts, rather than whole grains, legumes, vegetables, or fruits. The combination of increased consumption of refined grains and baked desserts, and decreased consumption of whole grains, legumes, fruits and vegetables, has led to America's obesity epidemic.

Fiber

Like starch, fiber is also a very large and complex molecule made up of anywhere from hundreds to thousands of smaller molecules strung together. Some of these molecules are glucose. Plants use fiber to form their skeletal or structural parts, such as stems. Our digestive system cannot break apart the bonds between the individual molecules in fiber. Therefore, even though fiber molecules contain glucose, we cannot use glucose or other molecules in fiber for energy. Hence, fiber provides no kilocalories to us. However, this zero kilocalorie nutrient is full of innumerable health benefits. It is very important to note that **fiber is only found in plant-based foods**. Many people don't realize that fiber is a type of carbohydrate and when they avoid grains, they lose out on the benefits of fiber. Here are some of the many benefits of fiber:[1]

- Lowers cholesterol by reducing the liver's production of cholesterol and by increasing intestinal elimination of cholesterol.
- Lowers the risk of diabetes by reducing the absorption of sugar and by reducing blood sugar levels.
- Improves colonic health. Fiber alleviates constipation, and reduces the risk of hemorrhoids, diverticular disease, and colon cancer.
- Reduces weight gain in several ways.
  - Foods that are naturally rich in fiber, such as whole grains, fruits, vegetables and legumes, are naturally low in sugar and fat, and are not as calorically dense as foods that do not have fiber, such as poultry, dairy, meat, or seafood.
  - Fiber also increases satiety, delays gastric emptying, attracts water, and slows the intestinal absorption of nutrients. Imagine fiber as very thin strands in our stomachs. These strands attract water and as the water fills our stomach, we feel full and eat less. These strands also reduce the speed at which food leaves our stomach, thereby leaving us feeling full longer.
  - Once the fiber enters our small intestines, where nutrients are absorbed, the fibrous strands delay the rate of nutrient absorption. When nutrients are absorbed quickly, their blood concentration rises quickly, and then falls quickly. The abrupt fall in blood concentration leads to hunger. However, when nutrients are absorbed slowly, their blood concentration rises gradually and stays elevated for a longer period of time, thereby leaving us feeling full longer.

- Fiber is a zero calorie food. Fiber provides tremendous health benefits without providing any calories.

Fiber is found naturally in all plant-based foods, and the type of fiber naturally found in food is known as dietary fiber. Fiber extracted from plant-based foods and then added to foods that do not naturally have fiber, is know as functional fiber. Food manufacturers often add fiber to cereals and bread made from refined grains. However, as we will see later when we discuss grains, foods made from whole grains are naturally rich in fiber.

Lactose

Lactose is a type of sugar found only in dairy products and it is less sweet than sucrose. Dairy milk has the most lactose content, followed by dairy yogurts and kefir. Lactose is what imparts a mildly sweet taste to plain dairy milk and yogurt. Most cheeses have very little lactose as most of the lactose is removed during cheese production. However, dairy products do not provide other nutrients found in plant-based foods such as fiber and anti-oxidants. Furthermore, as noted earlier, dairy consumption has been associated with type 1 diabetes, multiple sclerosis, and certain cancers. Dairy products are also high in fat and calories, thereby promoting weight gain.

**Whole Grains vs. Refined Grains**

Grains have been an essential part of the human diet for centuries and continue to remain an important part of the human diet. There are many different types of grains consumed around the world. Of all the carbohydrates, grains are the ones that lead to the most confusion because "low-carb" diets assert incorrectly that grains lead to weight gain.

Anatomy of a Grain

In order to understand the differences between refined and whole grains, let's review the anatomy of a grain. Generally speaking, grain kernels have three parts:[4]

1.  Bran is the outer thin layer. It contains most of the fiber, and many other nutrients, such as antioxidants, B vitamins, and phytochemicals, as well as minerals such as iron, copper, zinc, and magnesium.
2.  Endosperm is the bulk of the grain and it contains mostly starch, protein, and small amounts of some vitamins and minerals.
3.  Germ is the little seed inside the grain that can give rise to another new plant. It contains unsaturated fats, B vitamins, phytochemicals, and anti-oxidants like vitamin E.

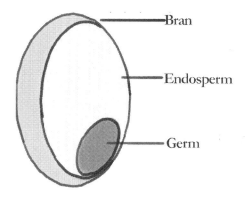

Whole grains contain all three parts of the grain in the proportion in which they are naturally found in the grain kernel. When grains are refined, the bran and germ are removed along with many other essential nutrients. You may have noticed the word "enriched" on many bread or pasta products. What does this mean? Since refining of grains leads to the loss of many key nutrients, Congress passed legislation in the early 1940s requiring that all grains that cross state lines be enriched with four vitamins and minerals: iron, thiamin, riboflavin, and niacin.[5] In 1996, folate was added to the list.[5] As Table 8-2 shows, enriching grain products with five nutrients still leaves many other nutrients lost during the refining process.[6,7]

### Table 8-2 How refining affects nutrients in wheat and rice

| Nutrient | Wheat (% of original nutrient remaining after refining) | Rice (% of original nutrient remaining after refining) | % of original nutrient after enrichment (wheat/rice) |
|---|---|---|---|
| Fiber | 25 | 37 | |
| Protein | 78 | 90 | |
| Calcium | 44 | | |
| Iron | 33 | 54 | 129 / 293 |
| Vitamin E | 8 | | |
| Vitamin B6 | 11 | 32 | |
| Vitamin K | 16 | 5 | |
| Magnesium | 16 | 17 | |
| Manganese | 17 | | |
| Zinc | 27 | | |
| Potassium | 29 | 52 | |
| Phosphorus | 30 | | |
| Copper | 35 | | |
| Selenium | 55 | | |
| Riboflavin (B2) | 24 | 53 | 299 (wheat) |
| Niacin (B3) | 25 | 31 | 119 / 82 |
| Thiamin (B1) | 24 | 17 | 156 / 144 |
| Folate | 59 | 40 | 661 / 1935 |

Whole grains are nutritious because they provide a combination of important nutrients, including fibers, starch, protein, healthy fats, vitamins, and minerals. On the other hand, refined grains provide mostly starch and protein and are devoid of many other key nutrients, such as fiber, vitamins, and minerals. In the past, people used to eat mostly whole grains. However, as our food supply became more industrialized, food manufacturers started using refined grains rather than whole grains. Why? Refined grains have a longer shelf life and their taste and texture is more appealing to consumers.[8] As food manufacturers have shifted from whole to refined grains, Americans have been consuming mostly refined grains. Whole grains are more filling than refined grains because they are rich in fiber and other nutrients that help us feel full. Therefore, we are more likely to eat a smaller volume of a whole grain food. On the other hand, because refined grains are devoid of most of the fiber and other nutrients, we are much more likely to feel less full and eat a larger quantity of the refined grains.

## Differentiating Whole from Refined Grains

How do you know whether the grains in the food you purchase are whole or refined? Certain gains, such as quinoa and oat, are always whole because it is not possible to remove their bran or seed. However, the bran and seed can be removed from many grains and they can be sold as refined or whole. When you purchase flours or other food items that contain grains, read the ingredient list. Generally speaking, if the word "whole" precedes the grain, then it is whole grain. Table 8-3 will also help you to determine whether the specific grains being used are whole or refined.[9]

## Table 8-3 How to differentiate whole and refined grains

| Grain | Whole if label says | Refined if label says |
|---|---|---|
| Amaranth | Always | |
| Barley | Hulled, Hull-less, Whole | Peal (bran is removed) |
| Buckwheat | Always | |
| Corn | Whole corn | Degermed |
| Kaniwa | Always | |
| Millet | Always | |
| Oats | Always | |
| Quinoa | Always | |
| Rice | Brown, Red, Black | White |
| Solid Rye | Whole rye or rye berries | |
| Rye Flours | Rey meal, pumpernickel | White rye, cream or light rye, medium rye, dark rye (maybe whole grain) |
| Sorghum | Usually whole grain, and definitely if the label says "whole sorghum" | |
| Teff | Always | |
| Triticale (hybrid of wheat and rye) | Almost always | |
| Wild Rice | Always | |

Oats are commonly sold as berries, steel/Irish cut oats, or rolled oats. Regardless of the form, they are always whole grains.[10] Oat berries are the actual oat kernels, which take a long time to boil and cook. Steel cut oats are oat berries that have been cut into smaller pieces, and this speeds the cooking process. Rolled oats have been partially cooked by steaming and then rolled flat. Since they are partially cooked, rolled oats cook the fastest.

## Wheat

You may have noticed that wheat isn't mentioned in Table 8-3. Wheat accounts for two-thirds of the grain eaten in the U.S.[11] However, most of the wheat in the U.S. is consumed in its refined form rather than whole form, usually as all-purpose flour in bread, pastas, and pizza dough.[11] There are many types of wheat available and depending upon the variety, it may or may not always be whole grain. All varieties of wheat contain gluten.[11] Table 8-4 outlines the various wheat varieties and how to differentiate whole from refined forms.[9]

## White Flour vs White Whole Wheat Flour[12]

Most of the wheat flour used in commercially-prepared breads, pastas, and baked goods is "white flour" or "all-purpose flour," which is refined wheat flour. On the other hand, "white whole wheat flour" is a whole grain flour made from white wheat that has a sweeter taste and milder texture than red whole wheat flour. Many recipes call for pastry flour, which is usually refined wheat flour. On the other hand, whole wheat pastry flour is white whole wheat flour and is therefore a whole grain. In our home, whenever a recipe calls for white or all-purpose flour, we substitute white whole wheat flour or whole wheat pastry flour.

## Table 8-4 Types of wheat

| Wheat | Whole grain if label says | Refined if label says | Notes |
|-------|---------------------------|-----------------------|-------|
| **Bulgur** | Always a whole grain | | Wheat kernels which are boiled, dried, cracked, then sorted by size and sold as fine or coarse. |
| **Durum** | Whole durum | Durum, semolina | Used for pastas and couscous |
| **Einkorn** | Always a whole grain | | |
| **Farro** | Whole Farro | Pearled farro | |
| **Flour** | "Whole wheat flour" or "100% whole wheat flour" | "Wheat" or "100% Wheat" | |
| **Kamut** | Whole kamut | Kamut | |
| **Red** | Whole red wheat | Red wheat | Heartier taste than white wheat |
| **Spelt** | Whole spelt | Spelt | Aka big farro or farro grande in Italy |
| **White** | Whole white wheat | White wheat | Milder and sweeter taste than red wheat |

## What about Gluten?

There has been considerable focus lately on gluten, and restaurants and grocery stores offer a variety of gluten-free products. What is gluten and do you need to avoid it? Gluten is a protein found primarily in wheat, barley, and rye. While the majority of the population tolerates gluten without any problems, some genetically predisposed individuals develop autoantibodies to gluten that then lead to celiac disease. Persons with celiac disease suffer from a variety of symptoms, such as chronic diarrhea and vitamin deficiencies, however some people have no symptoms at all.[13] A definitive diagnosis is made by blood tests, which detect autoantibodies, and with a biopsy of the small intestine.[14] The prevalence of celiac disease is approximately 1:70 to 1:300 in most countries.[13] Most persons with celiac disease need lifelong gluten-free diets.[15]

If you are concerned about celiac disease, it is best to see your physician for further evaluation. If you have already been diagnosed with celiac disease, it is best for you to follow closely with a physician and nutritionist or dietician who specializes in celiac disease.

Table 8-5 outlines which grains have gluten and which don't.[15,16]

## Table 8-5 Gluten content of grains

| Grain | Contains gluten |
|---|---|
| Amaranth | |
| Barley | Yes |
| Buckwheat | |
| Corn | |
| Millet | |
| Oats | Are gluten free in their pure form but can be contaminated with gluten; many experts advise limited amounts of oat intake in persons with mild celiac disease and complete avoidance in all others. |
| Quinoa | |
| Rice | Rice doesn't but brown rice syrup does |
| Rye | Yes |
| Sorghum | |
| Teff | |
| Triticale | Yes |
| Wheat (all types) | Yes |
| Wild Rice | No |

## Reading Nutrition Labels and Ingredients

In order to eat well, it is crucial to understand how to read nutrition and ingredient labels. Almost all commercially-sold foods are required to post ingredients and nutrition labels.

Ingredients

Regardless of what the food package claims, always read the ingredients list. When reading ingredients, keep in mind the following:

- The longer the list of ingredients, the more processed the food is.
- Ingredients are listed according to how much of the food they comprise. Ingredients which comprise the highest proportion of food are listed first, and the ingredient which comprises the least proportion of food is listed last.
- Determine whether or not any listed grain is whole or not.
- As I mentioned earlier, added sugars go by many different names, such as brown sugar, granulated sugar, powdered sugar, corn syrup, high fructose corn syrup, fructose, maple syrup, honey, agave, and juice concentrate.

Nutrition Labels

In this section, I will focus on the carbohydrates portion of the nutrition label. When reading a nutrition label, look for the following:

- Serving size and the amounts of servings per package. Sometimes they are one and the same, but most often there are two or more servings in a package.

- All of the information regarding calories, carbohydrates, fat, protein, vitamins, and minerals are for each serving size.
- Total carbohydrates include fiber, sugars, and starch.
  - Dietary fiber tells us the numbers of grams of fiber per serving.
  - Sugars tell us how many grams of sucrose or other sweeteners are there per serving. However, it doesn't tell us whether the sugars are naturally found in the food or added. The only way to tell if the food has added sugars is by reading the ingredients list.
  - Starch is not separated out in the carbohydrate section. However, if you take the total carbohydrates and subtract fiber and sugars from it, then you have the amount of starch in each serving.

## Nutrition and ingredient labels from a box of refined wheat pasta

INGREDIENTS: SEMOLINA, NIACIN, FERROUS SULFATE (IRON), THIAMINE MONONITRATE (VITAMIN B₁), RIBOFLAVIN (VITAMIN B₂) AND FOLIC ACID.
CONTAINS: WHEAT INGREDIENTS.

**Nutrition Facts**

Serving Size 5 Pieces (50g)
Servings Per Container 7

Amount Per Serving

Calories 200    Calories from Fat 10

| | % Daily Value* |
|---|---|
| **Total Fat** 1g | **2%** |
| Saturated Fat 0g | **0%** |
| *Trans* Fat 0g | |
| **Cholesterol** 0mg | **0%** |
| **Sodium** 0mg | **0%** |
| **Total Carbohydrate** 38g | **13%** |
| Dietary Fiber 2g | **6%** |
| Sugars 2g | |
| **Protein** 6g | |

| | | |
|---|---|---|
| Vitamin A 0% | • | Vitamin C 0% |
| Calcium 0% | • | Iron 10% |
| Thiamine 30% | • | Niacin 15% |
| Riboflavin 10% | • | Folic Acid 30% |

- The ingredients state semolina, which is durum flour. Since the label does not say whole semolina, it is refined flour.
- Since the pasta has been made from refined flour, fiber, vitamins, and minerals have been added back, per federal law.
- Each serving size is 50g and there are seven servings in the package.
- Each serving size has 38g of carbohydrates subdivided as follows:
  - Fiber 2g
  - Sugars 2g. Since the ingredients do not list sugar, we know the sugar in the pasta is from the sucrose naturally found in wheat.
  - Starch 34g

## Nutrition and ingredient labels from a box of whole wheat pasta

| **Nutrition Facts** | Amount Per Serving | % Daily Value* | Amount Per Serving | % Daily Value* |
|---|---|---|---|---|
| Serving Size 2 oz (56g) | **Total Fat** 1.5g | **2%** | **Total Carbohydrate** 39g | **13%** |
| Servings Per Container about 7 | Saturated Fat 0g | **0%** | Dietary Fiber 6g | **24%** |
| | Trans Fat 0g | | Soluble Fiber 1g | |
| | | | Insoluble Fiber 5g | |
| | **Cholesterol** 0mg | **0%** | Sugars 2g | |
| **Calories** 180 | **Sodium** 0mg | **0%** | **Protein** 8g | |
| Calories from Fat 15 | Iron 20% • Thiamin 15% • Niacin 25% • Folate 4% | | | |
| | Phosphorus 25% • Magnesium 20% • Manganese 80% | | | |

INGREDIENTS: WHOLE GRAIN DURUM WHEAT FLOUR.
CONTAINS WHEAT INGREDIENTS. THIS PRODUCT IS MANUFACTURED ON EQUIPMENT THAT PROCESSES PRODUCTS CONTAINING EGGS.

- The only ingredient is whole grain durum wheat flour, so we know it is whole grain pasta.
- Each serving size is 56g and there are seven servings in the entire package.
- Each serving size has 180 kcal.
- There are 39g of carbohydrates in each serving.
  - Of these, 6g are fiber.
  - 2g are from sugar. Since there is no sugar in the ingredient list, we know that these 2g are from the sucrose naturally found in wheat.
  - The remaining 31g are starch.

## Note: Nutritional content of whole wheat pasta vs. refined wheat pasta

- The whole wheat pasta and refined wheat pasta have comparable serving sizes (56g vs 50g).
- However, whole wheat pasta contains 6g of fiber vs. 2g in refined wheat pasta.
- Whole wheat pasta has 31g starch, whereas refined wheat pasta has 34g of starch.
- Whole wheat pasta is naturally rich in many vitamins and minerals such as iron, phosphorus, thiamin, magnesium, niacin, and manganese.
- However, most of the vitamins and minerals in refined wheat pasta were added to the flour after refining it.
- There are 8g of protein per serving of whole wheat pasta, but just 2g in refined wheat pasta.
- While a difference of 4g in fiber or 6g in protein may not seem like much, it important to remember that these differences are per serving and over the course of a day or week, the differences really add up.
- Though it may seem tempting to bridge the differences between the two pastas by adding more fiber or protein to the refined version, whole wheat pasta is naturally more nutritious than refined wheat pasta in all aspects. Further, it is very likely that whole grains offer hundreds of other nutrients that we haven't identified yet and that are likely lost through the refining process.

Summary of Carbohydrates

As I have outlined in this chapter, carbohydrates are a diverse group of nutrients that include sucrose, starch, fiber, and lactose. The key is to eat food groups that provide healthy carbohydrates. Fruits, vegetables, whole grains, and legumes are nutritionally dense as they provide ample fiber, vitamins, and nutrients with minimal sucrose. On the other hand, juices, sweetened beverages, desserts, and refined grains are nutritionally poor foods as they provide very little (if any) fiber, vitamins, and minerals, while providing a large quantity of sucrose. Carbohydrates got a bad rap because as our society has moved to more processed and commercially prepared foods, we have been eating more refined grains and more foods with large quantities of added sugars. It is no surprise then that increased consumption of nutritionally poor foods increased our rates of obesity and chronic diseases. Eating whole grains and fruits was never the problem. Rather, it was the increased consumption of refined grains, juices, sweetened beverages, and desserts.

Rather than eliminating whole grains or fruits as some fad diets recommend, it is more prudent to eliminate refined grains and added sugars. If there are times when you crave a sweet beverage, reach for water or fresh fruit and see if that satisfies your craving, as you may simply be thirsty or craving a refreshing sweet flavor. If you are still craving a sweet beverage, then try an occasional small serving of coconut juice, home made lemonade, or fresh squeezed orange or grapefruit juice. Table 8-6 provides a summary of healthy and unhealthy sources of carbohydrates.

## Table 8-6 Summary of carbohydrates

|  | Healthy | Avoid | Note |
|---|---|---|---|
| **Pasta** | Whole wheat pasta, orzo & couscous | Pastas that don't have the word "whole" preceding the wheat | Most pastas are made from wheat such as durum. |
| **Rice** | Brown, red, black rice | White rice | Wild rice is technically not a rice but a whole grain. |
| **Breads** | Breads made exclusively with whole grains | Breads made with refined grains | |
| **Tortillas** | Tortillas made with whole wheat or whole corn | Tortillas made from refined grains, degraded corn | |
| **Cereals** | Oats, bulgar, and cereals made with whole grains | Cereals made with refined grains; pre-sweetened oats; cream of wheat | |
| **Other grains** | Quinoa, bulgar, buckwheat, wild rice, millet | | |
| **Fruits** | All | Avoid fruit juices<br><br>Eat dried fruits in moderation as they are sweeter than the original fruit. Fruits are 90% water, and water is lost when the fruits are dried, thus making them sweeter. | |
| **Vegetables** | All | Fried vegetables | |
| **Legumes** | All | | |
| **Sweetened beverages** | Water is best to hydrate | Soda, sports drinks, juices, lemonade | |

## Special note about illness and whole grains

Whole grains are generally more nutritious than refined grains. However, there are times when we should eat refined grains instead. For example, when we contract a viral illness that leads to diarrhea, nausea, vomiting, loss of appetite, or abdominal pain. Another example is when patients are recovering from chemotherapy or anesthesia. In such instances, our digestive system is not working optimally and will not be able to digest whole grains adequately. Under these conditions, refined grains will be not only more palatable but also easier for our bodies to digest.

# Chapter 9
# **Fat and Cholesterol**

"Ghee" or clarified butter is commonly used in Indian cooking. Often considered a sign of affluence, a generous dollop of ghee is added to cooked lentils, vegetables, rice, and breads. I recently visited India after 14 years. While dining at a breakfast buffet, I asked the chef if one of the items was cooked with ghee. With his chest held up high, he replied a very proud yes. As I started to walk away, he asked me why I wasn't helping myself to the food item. When I told him that I don't eat ghee, he looked very perplexed and asked me why. I told him that it was for health reasons, and he seemed quite insulted. In a country where serving clarified butter to guests is synonymous with good hospitality, his reaction was understandable.

In this chapter, I will review how much fat we need to eat, the various types of fats, and the role fat and cholesterol play in our health. I will also review the fat and cholesterol content of various types of foods.

The food industry spends millions of dollars on research to figure out how to make food more appealing to consumers while minimizing production costs. As Pulitzer-Prize winning author Michael Moss explains in his book, *Salt Sugar Fat: How the Food Giants*

*Hooked Us*, three easy and inexpensive ways to make food tastier are by adding more sugar, fat, and salt.[1] Researchers know that sugar has something called a "bliss point," after which food tastes too sweet and consumers reject it.[1] But there is no bliss point for fat.[1] Industry researchers have learned that the more fat they add to a food, the more consumers like it.[1] Furthermore, adding sugar along with fat masks the richness of the food.[1] The food industry has used this information to sell foods that are very high in fat and sugar. Why is fat so appealing to our taste buds and what does fat taste like? Unlike sugar, salt, sour, or bitter, it is hard to define the taste of fat. Fatty foods have that creamy, melt-in-your-mouth feeling.[1] Research has shown that eating fat stimulates the pleasure centers in our brain.[1] If you eat a food and it "melts in your mouth," it very likely has a high fat content.

While fat is an essential component of a healthy diet, and fat and cholesterol play pivotal roles in our bodily functions, Americans are eating too much fat. Additionally, most people are eating the wrong types of fats. Not all fats are created equal. Some fats are beneficial while others are detrimental to our health. In this chapter, I will review how much fat we need to eat, the various types of fats, and the role fat and cholesterol play in our health. I will also review the fat and cholesterol content of various types of foods.

## Cholesterol

Do you know your cholesterol numbers? Your physician most likely checked them at your last physical. I find that most patients are interested in having their cholesterol checked, but very few know what cholesterol is, why we need it, how we get it, and which levels are cause for concern. In this section, I will review what cholesterol is, why our body needs it, how we get it, and the levels that are safe and unsafe.

Cholesterol and fat are often discussed together because they are both fat soluble molecules, i.e. they do not dissolve in water. Additionally, cholesterol-rich foods are often also rich in fat. While our body needs a certain amount of cholesterol, excess levels are detrimental.

There are two sources of cholesterol in our bodies: diet and endogenous production. Our livers can easily make cholesterol from other nutrients in our diet, and store it until needed. Therefore, cholesterol is not an essential nutrient, i.e. we do not need to consume it in our diet. It is important to note that **cholesterol is found in all animal-based foods. Cholesterol is not found in any plant-based foods.**

Our bodies need cholesterol for many important functions. Millions of cells in our bodies use cholesterol to build cell walls.[2] Other cells use cholesterol to synthesize sex hormones and vitamin D.[2] Our liver uses cholesterol to produce bile acids that help our small intestine digest and absorb fats.[2] Here is the important point: While we need some cholesterol, excess cholesterol is very harmful to our health, and significantly increases the risk of all cardiovascular diseases, such as heart attacks and strokes.

When physicians review cholesterol levels with their patients, they most likely mention "LDL cholesterol" and "HDL cholesterol." What do these phrases mean? The phrases "LDL" and "HDL" do not refer to different types of cholesterol, but rather the vehicles that carry cholesterol in our blood. Since cholesterol is fat soluble, it travels in our blood in special vehicles. While there are many such vehicles, the two that have been most widely studied and measured are low density lipoproteins (LDLs) and high density lipoproteins (HDLs). The total amount of cholesterol in our blood is a sum of the amount of cholesterol in different cholesterol-carrying vehicles.

**Breakdown of blood cholesterol**

Cholesterol in LDL
+ Cholesterol in HDL
+ Cholesterol in other vehicles
_____

**Total blood cholesterol**

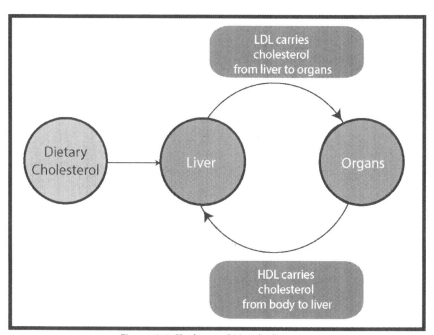

Figure 9-1 Cholesterol Metabolism

As illustrated in Figure 9-1, LDLs carry cholesterol away from the liver to the rest of our body, whereas HDLs remove cholesterol from various cells and return it to the liver. High levels of LDLs are especially harmful because excess cholesterol from LDLs is deposited into the blood vessels of our heart and brain, leading to dangerous blockages. In contrast, higher levels of HDLs are beneficial because HDLs are removing cholesterol from our blood vessels and other cells, and carrying it to the liver, from where it will eventually be excreted. We therefore want our LDL levels to be as low as possible, and our HDL levels to be as high as possible.

When you get your cholesterol levels checked, the laboratory measures the amount of total cholesterol and HDL cholesterol in you blood.[3] LDL cholesterol is then calculated using a special formula.[3] It is possible to measure the LDL cholesterol directly rather than calculating it. However, this is more expensive and is only done in situations when the calculated LDL values are likely to be inaccurate.[3]

Now that we have reviewed the different types of cholesterol measurements, what should your numbers be? Innumerable research studies have firmly established that there is a linear relationship between cholesterol levels and risk for coronary artery disease. As cholesterol levels increase, so does the risk of coronary artery disease. [4] The question then is at what cholesterol levels is our risk for heart disease the lowest, i.e. what is a safe cholesterol level? Most physicians base their recommendations on expert guidelines. However, the current guidelines are complex, controversial, and vary amongst the expert groups.[5,6,7] Most importantly, the "safe cholesterol" levels recommended by current guidelines are too high.[4] In order words, our cholesterol levels need to be much lower than considered acceptable by most guidelines.[4]

That conclusion is based on the findings of the Framingham Heart Study began, which began in 1948, and is an ongoing study under the direction of the National Heart, Lung, and Blood Institute and Boston University.[8] Framingham researchers have studied thousands of patients in order to investigate the risk factors associated with coronary artery disease. Framingham data show that only patients with total cholesterol levels less than 150 mg/dL have the lowest risk for cardiovascular disease.[4] In the first 50 years of the study, only five participants with total cholesterol less than 150 mg/dL developed coronary artery disease.[4] I rarely see patients with total cholesterol less than 150 mg/dL, as such low cholesterol levels are uncommon in the U.S. and other industrialized countries. However, rural populations in Asia, Africa, and Latin America usually have total cholesterol levels in the range of 125-140 mg/dL and they do not develop coronary artery disease.[4] Although many physicians and guidelines consider cholesterol levels between 150-200 to be "normal," 35% of coronary artery disease cases occur in people with total cholesterol levels in that range.[4]

What do the cholesterol numbers in America look like? Figures 9-2 and 9-3 show the cholesterol levels for adults according to a 2013 update from the American Heart Association (AHA).[9]

Figure 9-2: Americans with cholesterol > 200 mg/dL

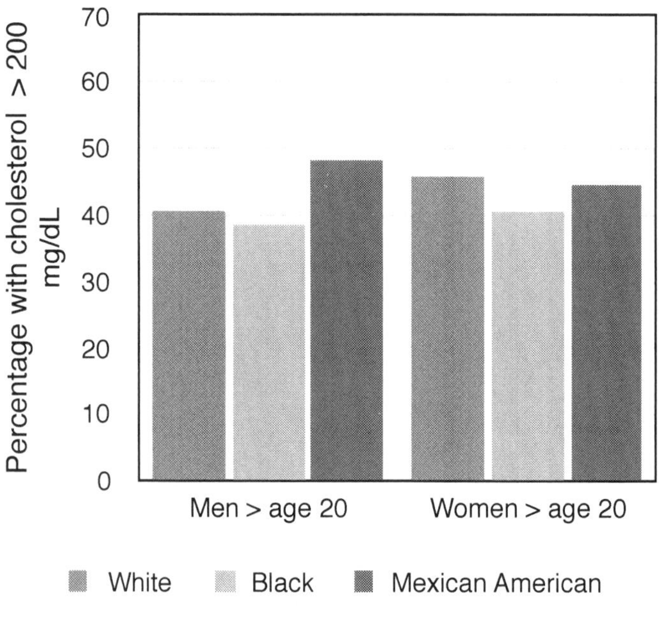

White     Black     Mexican American

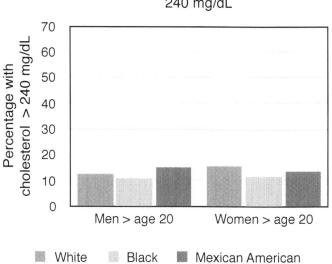

Figure 9-3: Americans with cholesterol >
240 mg/dL

As the AHA data show, the cholesterol numbers in America are much higher than those seen in rural populations in Asia, Africa, or Latin America. What has been considered "normal" cholesterol in the U.S. and other industrialized countries may actually represent high levels of mean cholesterol related to lifestyle and a primarily animal-based diet.

When evaluating cholesterol levels, another variable people should examine is the ratio of total cholesterol to HDL cholesterol. According to Framingham data, total cholesterol/HDL cholesterol ratios less than four are ideal. Ratios of total cholesterol to HDL cholesterol greater than four are associated with greater risk of coronary artery disease.[4]

### Table 9-1 Safe cholesterol levels

| Measurement | Safe |
| --- | --- |
| Total Cholesterol | < 150 mg/dL |
| Total cholesterol/HDL ratio | < 4 |

With every 1% reduction in LDL cholesterol, the risk of coronary artery disease falls by 2%.[4] The best way to achieve healthy cholesterol levels is to eat a whole-food, plant-based diet, exercise regularly, and maintain a healthy weight. Plant-based foods are naturally cholesterol free. In contrast, all animal-based foods contain significant amounts of cholesterol, thereby increasing cholesterol levels. Whole-food, plant-based diets are also rich in fiber, which helps our bodies excrete cholesterol. On the other hand, animal-based foods do not contain any fiber. Most animal-based foods also contain high levels of saturated fats, which increase LDL cholesterol levels, whereas most plant-based foods contain low levels of saturated fats. Tables 8-4 through 8-10 detail the cholesterol and saturated fat content of various plant and animal-based foods.

### Table 9-2 How plant- and animal-based foods affect cholesterol

| Food ingredient | Effect on cholesterol | Amount in plant-based foods | Amount in animal-based foods |
| --- | --- | --- | --- |
| Cholesterol | Increase | None | High |
| Fiber | Decrease | High | None |
| Saturated Fat | Increase LDL | Generally low | Generally high |

## Types of Dietary Fat

You have likely seen the terms "saturated fats," "trans fats," and "omega-3" used on food packages and in popular media. What do these terms mean and do you need to know them? In this section, I will review the various types of fats found in our foods and their impact on our health. I will also explain how to read food labels and evaluate the fat content of various types of foods.

Fats are very calorically dense as they provide nine calories per gram vs. four calories per gram of carbohydrates or proteins. The caloric density of fats is due to their complex chemical structure, comprised of carbon, oxygen, and hydrogen atoms. The configuration of hydrogen atoms in fats not only affects their chemical nature, but also their health impact. Dietary fats are subdivided into the following groups (Table 9-3) based upon the number of hydrogen atoms and their corresponding impact on our health.

- Saturated fats
- Monounsaturated and polyunsaturated fats
- Trans fats

## Table 9-3 Types of dietary fats

| Dietary Fat | Effect on cholesterol | Risk of cardio-vascular disease | Sources | Recommended daily amount |
|---|---|---|---|---|
| **Saturated** | Increase total cholesterol<br><br>Increase LDL | Increased | All animal-based foods, especially red meats and dairy<br><br>Plant-based foods: primarily cocoa, coconut, palm oil | Limit to less than 10% of daily calories |
| **Mono- & poly-unsaturated** | Decrease LDL | Maybe decreased | Animal-based foods: seafood, poultry, meat<br><br>Plant-based foods: nuts, seeds, various oils | Use in moderation |
| **Trans** | Increase LDL<br><br>Reduce HDL | Increased | Commercially-prepared pastries and deep-fried foods<br><br>Some margarines | Avoid completely |

Saturated Fats

Saturated fats contain as many hydrogen atoms as chemically possible. In other words, the molecules are "saturated" with hydrogen atoms that directly impact their physical and biological properties. Due to their chemical structure, saturated fats are solid at room temperature. For example, butter and coconut oil contain a high amount of saturated fat.

Saturated fats have many deleterious effects on our bodies:[10-12]

- Increase total cholesterol and LDL (bad) cholesterol
- Increase risk for cardiovascular disease
- Increase risk of cancer
- Increase risk for dementia

Saturated fats are found in almost all animal-based foods. While the amount of saturated fats is greatest in red meats and dairy products, they are also found in poultry, eggs, and seafood. Most plant-based foods have minimal amounts of saturated fats with the exception of cocoa, palm oil, and coconut oil.

Monounsaturated and Polyunsaturated Fats

Monounsaturated and polyunsaturated fats are not saturated with hydrogen atoms. Monounsaturated fats are missing two hydrogen atoms, whereas polyunsaturated fats are missing four or more hydrogen atoms. As a result of the missing atoms, both types of unsaturated fats are liquids at room temperature. For example, vegetable oils are liquids at room temperature because most of their fats are monounsaturated and polyunsaturated.

Monounsaturated and polyunsaturated fats are generally healthier than saturated fats as they both lower our LDL (bad) cholesterol and may reduce the risk of heart disease.[10] Except for the saturated fats founds in cocoa, coconut and palm oil, most of the fats in plant-based foods are monounsaturated and polyunsaturated fats. Fatty fish are the primary source of unsaturated fats in animal-based foods, though smaller amounts are found in meat, dairy, and poultry.

**Table 9-4 Sources of monounsaturated and polyunsaturated fats**

| Plant-based foods[10] | Animal-based foods[10] |
| --- | --- |
| Nuts | Fatty fish |
| Seeds | Meat: small amount |
| Avocados | Poultry: small amount |
| Olives | |
| Oils: canola, olive, vegetable | |

You may have heard of food manufacturers or various diet experts touting the benefits of omega-3 or omega-6 fats. What are these? While it is not important to know the specifics, I am reviewing them here for completeness. Omega-3 and omega-6 are types of polyunsaturated fats. The nomenclature "omega 3" or "omega 6" refers to the location where some of the hydrogen atoms are missing in these polyunsaturated fats. Linoleic acid is a type of omega-6 fat, and linolenic acid is a type of omega-3 fat. Both linoleic and linolenic acids are essential fats because our bodies cannot synthesize them, and we must consume them in our diet. However, it is not necessary to take supplements of either as both can be easily consumed through a wide variety of plant- and animal-based foods:

- Linoleic acid (omega-6) found in vegetable oils (corn, sunflower, safflower, soybean, cottonseed), nuts, seeds, poultry fat
- Linolenic acid (omega-3) found in oils (flaxseed, canola, walnut, wheat germ, soybean), nuts and seeds, soybeans, seafood

## Trans Fats

You have likely heard of trans fats and that they should be avoided. What exactly are they and why are they bad for us? Trans fats were created by the food industry because they are easier to cook with and spoil less easily than natural fats. To produce trans fats, hydrogen atoms are added to mono or polyunsaturated fats. The process of adding hydrogen atoms to unsaturated fats is known as hydrogenation. Doing so improves the texture and taste of foods. For example, margarines become more spreadable, pastries more flaky, and puddings more creamy.

Some trans fats are found naturally in animal-based foods such as dairy products and red meat. However, the majority of the trans fats we eat are a product of industrial hydrogenation. Most Americans consume trans fats in commercially-prepared foods such as:[2,10]

- Certain margarines
- Cookies, cakes, pies, and other pastries
- Commercially deep-fried foods

Trans fats are particularly detrimental to health because they have been shown to:[2,10]

- Increase LDL (bad) cholesterol
- Decrease HDL (good) cholesterol
- Increase the risk of cardiovascular disease
- Interfere with the health benefits of polyunsaturated fats

How do you know whether the food you are eating contains trans fats? By checking the nutrition label or reviewing the ingredients list. If the purchased food comes with a nutrition label, the easiest thing to do is to check for trans fats in the nutrition label. In 2006, the FDA began to require that all nutrition labels indicate the trans fat content of foods.[13] However, foods that contain less than 0.5g of trans fat per serving may claim trans fats content as zero in the nutrition label.[13] Therefore, it is also important to read the ingredients list. When evaluating the ingredients list, look for the words "partially hydrogenated" or "hydrogenated," which indicate the presence of trans fats.[2,10]

In 2015, the FDA announced that trans fats are "generally recognized as unsafe," and required food manufacturers to remove all trans fats from foods. Food manufacturers will have three years to comply with the requirement.[13]

## How Much Fat Do We Need?

After reviewing the various types of dietary fat and their health effects, you are most likely wondering how much saturated, unsaturated, and total fat you should eat each day. We need some fat in our diets since fat serves several essential functions in our bodies. It provides cushioning, thermoregulation, and energy in times of starvation. Many hormones are made from fats. The millions of cells in our bodies use fat molecules to build their cell walls.

According to research data from the China study, people in China consumed 14.5% of their daily calories from fat (compared to 34-38% for Americans) and had far lower rates of cardiovascular disease, cancer, and other chronic diseases.[14] Furthermore, Drs. Dean Ornish and Caldwell Esselstyn both reversed coronary heart disease in their patients using low-fat diets. The patients in their studies consumed approximately 10% of their daily calories from fat.[15-19] Based upon the results of the aforementioned studies:

- Most adults should limit their daily fat intake to about 10% of total calories.

- Most of our fat calories should be in the form of monounsaturated and polyunsaturated fats found in plant-based foods.
- We should limit the amounts of saturated fats found in cocoa, palm oil, and coconut.
- We should avoid trans fats completely as they worsen our cholesterol profiles and increase the risk of developing heart disease.
- We should avoid all animal-based foods as they contain significant amounts of saturated fat, cholesterol, and carcinogens.

Unfortunately, most Americans are consuming far more than 10% of their daily calories from fat. According to the Centers for Disease Control and Prevention:[20]

- American men consume 33.6% of their daily calories from fat and 11% of their daily calories from saturated fats.
- American women consume 33.5% of their daily calories from fat and 11% of their daily calories from saturated fat.

There are several reasons why Americans are consuming far more fat than advisable. First, the food industry and restaurants use a large amount of fat when preparing food in order to enhance its flavor and appeal. Second, the American diet is heavily based on animal-based foods, which contain a large amount of fat. Third, most health care providers recommend high levels of fat intake based on dietary guidelines that have not kept pace with nutrition research. By law, the U.S. Department of Agriculture and the U.S. Department of Health and Human Services issue joint "Dietary Guidelines for Americans" every five years. The latest guidelines that were released in January 2016 reported the following findings and recommendations:[21]

- Most Americans exceed the recommended amounts of sodium, refined grains, added sugars, and saturated fats.
- Most Americans do not consume enough fruits, vegetables, and whole grains.
- Americans should limit the intake of saturated fat to <10% of daily calories.
- Americans should consume no more than 10% of daily calories from added sugars.
- The 2010 guidelines advised limiting daily cholesterol intake to less than 300mg/day. Guidelines issued in 2016 did not state an upper limit on dietary cholesterol intake but made the following recommendations:
  - "As recommended by the [Institute of Medicine], individuals should eat as little dietary cholesterol as possible while consuming a healthy eating pattern. In general, foods that are higher in dietary cholesterol, such as fatty meats and high-fat dairy products, are also higher in saturated fats."[21]
  - "Strong evidence from mostly prospective cohort studies but also randomized controlled trials has shown that eating patterns that include lower intake of dietary cholesterol are associated with reduced risk of CVD, and moderate evidence indicates that these eating patterns are associated with reduced risk of obesity."[21]
  - "Dietary cholesterol is found only in animal foods such as egg yolk, dairy products, shellfish, meats, and poultry. A few foods, notably egg yolks and some shellfish, are higher in dietary cholesterol but not saturated fats."[21]
- The 2010 guidelines recommended limiting total fat intake to 20-35% of daily calories. This upper limit was removed from the latest guidelines.

The guidelines released in 2016 have taken some steps forward by advising consumers to limit their intake of added sugars, saturated fat, and dietary cholesterol. However, the guidelines have taken a major step backwards by removing the upper limits on fat and cholesterol intake. Unfortunately, this has prompted some "low-carb" proponents to erroneously claim that dietary cholesterol does not matter, and that high-fat diets are healthy for us.

## Fat and Cholesterol Content of Various Foods

In the following pages and tables, we will review the amount and types of fats found in various plant- and animal-based foods. For each food item, I have listed the amount of total and saturated fat. The difference between the two equals the amount of mono and polyunsaturated fats. As we review the fat content of different foods, notice the following generalizations:

- All plant-based foods are cholesterol free whereas all animal-based foods contain cholesterol.
- Fruits and vegetables have negligible amounts of fat.
- Whole grains and legumes provide minimal amounts of fat.
- The primary sources of fats in plant-based fats are soy products, avocados, cocoa, coconut, nuts, seeds, olives, and vegetable oils.
- With the exception of cocoa, coconut, and palm oil, the majority of fats in plant-based foods are mono and polyunsaturated fats.
- Red meats, poultry, and dairy have high levels of total and saturated fat.
- Even animal-based foods with minimal fat content, such as shrimp, deliver significant amounts of cholesterol.

Table 9-5 Fat and cholesterol content of fruits & vegetables

| Per Serving | Size | Total calories | Fat calories | % calories from fat | Total fat (g) | Saturated fat (g) | Cholesterol (mg) |
|---|---|---|---|---|---|---|---|
| Bananas | 1 peeled banana | 105 | 3.6 | 3.4% | 0.4g | 0.1g | 0 |
| Grapes | 1/2 cup | 52 | 0.9 | 1.7% | 0.1g | 0 | 0 |
| Apples | 1 apple (138g) | 72 | 1.8 | 2.5% | 0.2g | 0 | 0 |
| Oranges | 1 orange (131g) | 62 | 1.8 | 3% | 0.2g | 0 | 0 |
| Tomatoes | 1 tomato (123g) | 22 | 1.8 | 8% | 0.2 | 0 | 0 |
| Peas | 2/3 cup | 70 | 0 | 0 | 0 | 0 | 0 |
| Green beans | 2/3 cup | 30 | 0 | 0 | 0 | 0 | 0 |
| Carrots | 8 baby carrots | 28 | 0.9 | 3.2% | 0.1g | 0 | 0 |
| Potatoes | 1 potato (202g) | 188 | 2.7 | 1.4% | 0.3g | 0.1g | 0 |
| Spinach | 1 cup (30g) | 7 | 0.9 | 13% | 0.1g | 0 | 0 |
| Avocado | 1/2 cup | 192 | 159 | 83% | 17.7g | 2.4g | 0 |

As Table 9-5 shows, most fruits and vegetables provide a negligible amount of fat per serving. You may have noticed that 13% of the calories in spinach are from fat, which may seem high compared to other fruits and vegetables. However, the overall fat content of one cup of spinach is very low, as it contains only 0.9g of fat. Avocados are unique amongst vegetables in that a large proportion of their calories are from fat. Of the 17.7g of fat in half a cup of avocado, only 2.4g are from saturated fat. Therefore, most the the fat in avocados is mono and polyunsaturated. Due to their high fat content, avocados should be consumed in modest amounts.

Whole grains and legumes are generally low in fat, providing about 5-17% of calories from fat (Table 9-6). Additionally they are low in saturated fat. I have included tofu and soy milk in this table because they are made from soybeans, which are a type of legume. Unlike other legumes, soybeans, and subsequently tofu and soy milk, provide a fair amount of fat per serving. Fortunately, very little of the fat is saturated and most of it is mono and polyunsaturated.

Table 9-6 Fat and cholesterol content of whole grains & legumes

| Per Serving | Size | Total calories | Fat calories | % calories from fat | Total fat (g) | Saturated fat (g) | Cholesterol (mg) |
|---|---|---|---|---|---|---|---|
| Whole wheat pasta | 2oz dry | 200 | 10 | 5% | 1g | 0 | 0 |
| Brown rice | 1/4 cup dry | 180 | 15 | 8% | 1.5g | 0 | 0 |
| Quinoa | 1oz dry | 100 | 15 | 15% | 1.5g | 0 | 0 |
| Irish oatmeal | 1/4 cup dry | 150 | 25 | 17% | 2.5g | 0.5g | 0 |
| Black beans | 1/2 cup cooked | 110 | 0 | 0 | 0 | 0 | 0 |
| Pinto beans | 1/4 cup dry | 100 | 5 | 5% | 0.5g | 0 | 0 |
| Garbanzo beans | 1/4 cup dry | 180 | 25 | 14% | 3g | 0 | 0 |
| Tofu | 3 oz | 80 | 35 | 44% | 4g | 0.5g | 0 |
| Soymilk | 1 cup | 80 | 35 | 44% | 4g | 0.5g | 0 |

Most of the calories in nuts, seeds, coconut, and cocoa are from fat, as seen in Table 9-7. With the exception of cocoa and coconut, saturated fat comprises a small portion of the fat. Coconut and cocoa do provide a fair amount of saturated fat. Not surprisingly, all of the calories in vegetable oils and margarine are from fat. In contrast to butter, the majority of fat in plant-based margarine is not saturated. Due to their high fat content, nuts, seeds, coconut, and cocoa should be consumed in moderation. Additionally, we should minimize the use of added oils in cooking, garnishing, seasoning, etc.

### Table 9-7 Plant-based foods with high amounts of fat

| Per Serving | Serving size | Total calories | Fat Calories | % calories from fat | Total fat (g) | Saturated fat (g) | Cholesterol (mg) |
|---|---|---|---|---|---|---|---|
| 100% Cocoa | 1 Tbsp | 20 | 10 | 50% | 1.5g | 0.5g | 0 |
| Coconut | 3 Tbsp | 120 | 100 | 83% | 11g | 10g | 0 |
| Avocado | 1/2 cup | 192 | 159 | 83% | 17.7g | 2.4g | 0 |
| Walnuts | 1/4 cup | 190 | 170 | 89% | 18g | 1.5g | 0 |
| Almonds | 1/3 cup | 160 | 130 | 81% | 14g | 1g | 0 |
| Roasted peanuts | 1/4 cup | 170 | 130 | 76% | 15g | 2.5g | 0 |
| Flax seeds | 1/4 cup | 225 | 159 | 71% | 17.7g | 1.7g | 0 |
| Canola oil | 1 Tbsp | 120 | 120 | 100% | 14g | 1g | 0 |
| Olive oil | 1 Tbsp | 120 | 120 | 100% | 14g | 2g | 0 |
| Plant-based margarine | 1 Tbsp | 100 | 100 | 100% | 11g | 3 | 0 |

Table 9-8 Fat and cholesterol content of dairy products

| Per Serving | Serving size | Total calories | Fat Calories | % calories from fat | Total fat (g) | Saturated fat (g) | Cholesterol (mg) |
|---|---|---|---|---|---|---|---|
| Whole dairy milk | 1 cup | 150 | 70 | 47% | 8g | 4.5g | 25mg |
| 2% fat dairy milk | 1 cup | 120 | 45 | 38% | 5g | 3g | 20mg |
| 1% fat dairy milk | 1 cup | 100 | 22 | 22% | 2g | 1.5g | 9mg |
| Whole milk plain yogurt | 1 cup | 170 | 80 | 47% | 9g | 5g | 35mg |
| Low-fat plain yogurt | 1 cup | 120 | 20 | 17% | 2g | 1.5g | 15mg |
| 1% milk fat peach dairy yogurt | 1 individual size container | 130 | 15 | 12% | 1.5g | 1g | 10mg |
| Cheddar cheese | 1 oz. | 110 | 80 | 73% | 9g | 5g | 30mg |
| Mozzarella cheese | ¼ cup | 90 | 60 | 67% | 7g | 4.5g | 25mg |
| Butter | 1 Tbsp | 100 | 100 | 100% | 11g | 7g | 30mg |

Dairy products are rich in total and saturated fat. When analyzing the fat content of dairy products, it is important to look at the percentage of calories from fat (Table 9-8). The dairy industry lists the fat content of its products as a percentage of weight rather than calories. For example, whole milk is 4% fat by weight. However 47% of the calories in whole milk are from fat. Similarly, the percentage of calories from fat in 2% and 1% milk are 38% and 22%, respectively. Most of the calories in cheese are form fat, especially saturated fat. Additionally, cheese, along with all dairy products, provides a fair amount of cholesterol.

Americans now consume over 33 pounds of cheese or cheese-type products per year, triple the amount eaten in the 1970s.[1] Thirty three pounds of cheese provide 60,000 calories and 3,100 grams of saturated fat. If the average person eats 2,000 calories per day, then 60,000 calories are enough to sustain the average person for 30 days. Cheese accounts for the largest source of saturated fat in the American diet.[1]

As we see in the Table 9-9, red meats are very high in total and saturated fat, with the majority of calories from fat. The high fat content of red meat also makes it very calorically dense. Additionally, red meats have high levels of cholesterol. It is important to note that the serving size in the above table is four ounces of red meat. But most restaurant and home serving sizes are significantly larger. Pork is often advertised as a white meat by the pork industry. From a nutrition perspective, pork is a red meat, with a similar fat and cholesterol profile as other red meats.[22,23] As mentioned earlier in Chapter 2, the World Health Organization has recently concluded that the consumption of red meat likely contributes to the onset of cancer.

#### Table 9-9 Fat and cholesterol content of red meats

| Per Serving | Serving size | Total calories | Fat Calories | % calories from fat | Total fat (g) | Saturated fat (g) | Cholesterol (mg) |
|---|---|---|---|---|---|---|---|
| Lamb loin chop | 4 oz | 350 | 270 | 77% | 30g | 13g | 85mg |
| Angus beef steak | 4 oz | 200 | 110 | 55% | 12g | 5g | 60mg |
| Beef burger patty | 1 patty (151g) | 325 | 200 | 62% | 23g | 10g | 105mg |
| Beef hot dog | 1 link (53g) | 160 | 130 | 81% | 15g | 6g | 30mg |
| Pork | 4 oz | 220 | 130 | 59% | 14g | 5g | 75mg |
| Black Forest ham | 2 oz | 50 | 15 | 30% | 1.5g | 0.5g | 20mg |

Many people believe that chicken and other poultry foods are healthy. However, as shown in Table 9-10, poultry items are also rich in total and saturated fat. Almost half of the calories in poultry are from fat, and all poultry foods have high levels of cholesterol. For example, one egg delivers 210mg of cholesterol. And all processed meats, including those from poultry, contribute to the onset of cancer according to the recent WHO report.[22,23]

### Table 9-10 Fat and cholesterol in poultry foods

| Per Serving | Serving size | Total calories | Fat calories | % calories from fat | Total fat (g) | Saturated fat (g) | Cholesterol (mg) |
|---|---|---|---|---|---|---|---|
| Eggs | 1 egg (50g) | 60 | 35 | 58% | 4g | 1.5g | 210mg |
| Boneless skinless chicken thigh | 4 oz | 160 | 70 | 44% | 8g | 2.5g | 70mg |
| Chicken with skin | 4 oz | 200 | 100 | 50% | 12g | 4g | 65mg |
| Chicken nuggets | 7 nuggets (88g) | 180 | 80 | 44% | 9g | 2g | 35mg |
| Ground Turkey | 4 oz | 170 | 80 | 47% | 9g | 2.5g | 85mg |

Table 9-11 Fat and cholesterol in seafood

| Per Serving | Serving size | Total calories | Fat Calories | % calories from fat | Total fat (g) | Saturated fat (g) | Cholesterol (mg) |
|---|---|---|---|---|---|---|---|
| **Raw shrimp** | 4 oz | 100 | 5 | 5% | 0.5g | 0 | 135mg |
| **Yellow fin tuna** | 6 oz | 210 | 25 | 12% | 2.5g | 0 | 90mg |
| **Smoked salmon** | 2 oz | 70 | 20 | 29% | 2.5g | 0.5g | 30mg |

Although seafood has less total and saturated fat than other animal-based foods (Table 9-11), it contains a fair amount of cholesterol. For example, a four-ounce serving of shrimp contains no fat but delivers 135mg of cholesterol. As with other meats, seafood contains several known carcinogens, such as heterocyclic amines (HCA) and polycyclic aromatic hydrocarbons (PAH), which are formed during processing or cooking.[24]

# Reading food labels - butter vs. margarine

Dairy butter

Plant-based margarine

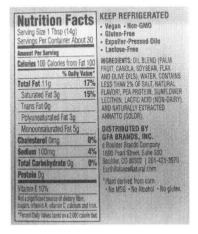

- The label on the left is for butter and the label on the right is for plant-based margarine
- Both have the same serving size of 1 Tbsp (14g)
- Both have total fat of 11g per serving
- Butter has 7g of saturated fat per serving whereas plant-based margarine has 3g.
- Since most of the fat in butter is saturated, butter is solid at room temperature.
- Margarine is semi-solid at room temperature because most of its fat is mono and polyunsaturated.
- Butter has 30mg of cholesterol per serving whereas the margarine has none.
- Neither provide any carbohydrates or protein or trans fats.
- When selecting a margarine, it is very important to read the ingredients list to look for the words, "hydrogenated" or "partially hydrogenated." Since these words are not listed, the margarine does not have any trans fats, which is also confirmed in the nutrition label.

# Chapter 10
# Why Protein Is Not Always the Answer

There are many common misconceptions regarding protein. For years, low-carb, high protein diets have been telling people that they are not eating enough protein, and that eating more protein will help them lose weight. The message has been further perpetuated by an opportunistic food industry advertising high levels of protein in various animal-based and processed foods. It's also said that a plant-based diet will not provide adequate amounts of protein, and that it is essential to eat animal-based foods in order to get enough protein. However, the human body needs far less protein than most people believe. Excess protein isn't always beneficial and can even be harmful. In this chapter, I will review the role proteins play in our health, our daily protein requirements, as well as healthy sources of protein.

## What Are Proteins and Why Do We Need Them?

Proteins are long complex molecules made up of amino acids. Think of amino acids as the building blocks for proteins. There are 20 amino acids, of which nine are essential.[1] The word "essential" means that our bodies cannot make the nine essential amino acids, and we must consume them in our diet. The remaining 11 amino acids can be synthesized by our bodies. Tens to hundreds of amino acids are connected in uniques sequences and shapes to build specific proteins.

When most people think of proteins, they think of skeletal muscles. However, there is a lot more to proteins, which are involved in virtually every function in the human body. Here are some of the many roles proteins play:[1]

- They are used as basic building material for most structures, such as skin, muscle, bone, tendons, organs, blood, etc.
- They facilitate millions of crucial reactions in our bodies every day.
- They carry important molecules in our blood or within our cells. (Hemoglobin is a very complex protein that carries oxygen in our blood.)
- They become antibodies, which are crucial in fighting infections.
- They are the foundation of many hormones.
- They work as neurotransmitters, which help nerve endings communicate with one another.
- They act as buffers for acids and bases.
- They help regulate fluid balance.
- They are used for energy in times of starvation.

When we consume dietary proteins, our digestive system breaks the proteins into their individual amino acids, and then absorbs them.

Our bodies then reassemble the amino acids into various proteins to replenish damaged or needed proteins. Excess amino acids are subsequently converted to fat and stored as such. Contrary to popular belief, consuming excess protein will not increase our muscle size or strength. Only regular physical exercise can do so.[1]

While proteins serve important functions, and a deficiency can lead to serious health problems, excess protein consumption can also be problematic.

- High-protein diets lead to calcium wasting in the urine, which increases the risk for osteoporosis.[1,2]
- All amino acids contain nitrogen. Any unneeded nitrogen is cleared by the kidneys, and excess protein consumption places an additional burden on the kidneys. High-protein diets can worsen kidney function in people with pre-existing kidney disease.[1,2]
- Most individuals who consume high levels of protein do so from animal-based foods such as dairy, red meat, and poultry. As I have reviewed previously, animal-based foods are very high in fat and do not provide any fiber. Furthermore, there is definitive research linking animal-based foods with cardiovascular disease and cancer. It is much more difficult to consume excess amounts of protein from a plant-based diet.

Many popular "low-carb" fad diets advocate eating high amounts of protein while minimizing carbohydrates, i.e. grains. When people start such diets, they usually do see an immediate weight loss. However, the weight loss is due to overall reduction of calories from not eating grains, and due to water loss.[1,2] When we consume more protein than we need, we are also consuming an excess amount of nitrogen. Our kidneys then excrete the extra nitrogen along with water in the form of urine. The water loss in turn contributes to weight loss. While such diets work for a short period of time, they rarely lead to long-term weight loss due to the unpalatability of a low-grain diet. Meals without grains, such as rice, pasta, or breads, are not enjoyable or satisfying. Additionally, high-protein diets are harmful in the long term because they are high in animal-based foods and low in nutritious whole grains.

## How Much Protein Do We Need?

Humans need far less protein than commonly believed. The recommended daily allowance (RDA) for adults is 0.8g/kg/day.[1,2] RDA values are higher during pregnancy, lactation, and for young children. For an average 70 kg (154 lb.) adult, the RDA would be calculated as follows:

$$70 \text{ kg} \times (.8\text{g/kg/day}) = 56 \text{ g of protein/day}$$

One gram of protein provides four calories. For an average 70 kg person consuming 2,000 calories per day, 56g of protein would equate to 224 calories or 11% of daily calories. We only need to consume roughly 11% of daily calories from protein.

While most Americans are concerned that they are not eating enough protein, research data show otherwise. The National Health and Nutrition Examination Survey (NHANES) is the primary source of nutritional data in the U.S. NHANES data from 2011-2012 regarding the daily protein consumption by adults are shown in Table 10-1.[3]

**Table 10-1 Daily mean protein consumption by American men & women**

| Age | Men - Mean daily protein consumption in grams | Women - Mean daily protein consumption in grams |
| --- | --- | --- |
| 20-29 | 102.9 | 72.1 |
| 30-39 | 110.0 | 75.5 |
| 40-49 | 104.8 | 66.4 |
| 50-59 | 95.2 | 68.0 |
| 60-69 | 89.7 | 65.2 |
| 70 or greater | 80 | 58.8 |

As we see in Table 10-1, most Americans are consuming far more protein than they need. Why then is there such a disparity between how much protein people think they need and how much they are actually consuming? There are two main reasons. First, popular fad diets have been erroneously telling consumers that they are not eating enough protein and that eating more protein will help them lose weight. Second, while 56g of proteins for an average 70 kg adult may seem like a lot, it is very easy to consume this amount from a variety of foods, as outlined in the next section.

## How Much Protein Is in the Foods We Eat?

Notwithstanding popular belief, it is easy to consume an adequate amount of protein every day. A variety of plant- and animal-based foods provide ample protein for our daily needs as shown in Tables 10-2 and 10-3.

## Table 10-2 Protein in various animal-based foods

| Per Serving | Serving size | Protein (g) | Total calories | Calories from protein | % calories from protein | Fat (g) | Choles-terol (mg) | Fiber (g) |
|---|---|---|---|---|---|---|---|---|
| Dairy Milk 1% fat | 1 cup | 8g | 110 | 32 | 29% | 2.5g | 15mg | 0 |
| Low-fat peach dairy yogurt | 1 cup | 7g | 130 | 28 | 22% | 1.5g | 10mg | 0 |
| Cheddar cheese | 1 oz. | 7g | 110 | 28 | 25% | 9g | 30mg | 0 |
| Eggs | 1 egg (50g) | 6g | 60 | 24 | 40% | 4g | 210mg | 0 |
| Chicken | boneless 1/2 breast (145g) | 30.23g | 249 | 121 | 49% | 13g | 93mg | 0 |
| Chicken nuggets | 7 nuggets (88g) | 12g | 180 | 48 | 27% | 9g | 35mg | 0 |
| Smoked salmon | 2 oz | 13g | 70 | 52 | 74% | 1.5g | 10mg | 0 |
| Filet Mignon | 5 oz | 28g | 350 | 112 | 32% | 25g | 90mg | 0 |
| Beef burger patty | 1 patty (151g) | 26g | 325 | 104 | 32% | 23g | 105mg | 0 |

## Table 10-3 Protein in various plant-based foods

| Per Serving | Serving size | Protein (g) | Total calories | Calories from protein | % calories from protein | Fat (g) | Choles-terol (mg) | Fiber (g) |
|---|---|---|---|---|---|---|---|---|
| Orange | 1 fresh orange | 1.2g | 62 | 4.8 | 8% | 0.2g | 0 | 3.1g |
| Apple | 1 raw apple with peel | 0.4g | 72 | 1.6 | 2.2% | 0.2g | 0 | 3.3g |
| Green beans | 2/3 cup | 1g | 30 | 4 | 13% | 0 | 0 | 2g |
| Peas | 2/3 cup | 4g | 70 | 16 | 23% | 0 | 0 | 4g |
| Spinach | 1 cup raw chopped | 0.9g | 7 | 3.6 | 51% | 0.1g | 0 | 0.7g |
| Steel cut oats | 1/4 cup dry | 4g | 150 | 16 | 11% | 2.5g | 0 | 3g |
| Whole wheat pasta | 2 oz dry pasta | 7g | 180 | 28 | 16% | 1g | 0 | 6g |
| Whole wheat burger buns | 1 bun | 6g | 140 | 24 | 17% | 2g | 0 | 4g |
| Brown rice | 1/4 cup dry rice | 4g | 150 | 16 | 11% | 1.5g | 0 | 2g |
| Quinoa | 1oz dry | 4g | 100 | 16 | 16% | 1.5g | 0 | 2g |
| Peanut butter | 2 TBSP (32g) | 9g | 180 | 36 | 20% | 16g | 0 | 1g |
| Black beans | 1/2 cup cooked | 7g | 110 | 28 | 25% | 0 | 0 | 7g |
| Chick Peas | 1/4 cup dry | 10g | 180 | 40 | 22% | 3g | 0 | 9g |
| Tofu | 3 oz | 9g | 80 | 36 | 45% | 4g | 0 | 1g |
| Soymilk | 1 cup | 7g | 80 | 28 | 35% | 4g | 0 | 2g |

As seen in Table 10-3, plant-based foods provide variable amounts of protein. When assessing the protein content of various plant-based foods, we can make the following generalizations (though there are notable exceptions):

- Fruits - provide minimal amounts of protein.
- Vegetables - about 10% of the calories are from protein though some, like spinach, provide 50% of calories from protein.
- Whole grains - about 10% of the calories are from protein.
- Legumes and Beans - about 30% of the calories are from protein.
- Soybeans, tofu, soy milk - about 30% of the calories are from protein.

In addition to providing enough protein, plant-based foods have other health benefits. They are naturally cholesterol free, low in fat (except for nuts, olives, cocoa, and avocado), and high in fiber. Additionally, consuming a whole-food, plant-based diet reduces the risk of most chronic diseases.

As we can see in Table 10-2 and 10-3, animal-based foods provide a sizable amount of protein per serving. Since animal-based foods account for a large share of the calories consumed by Americans, it is easy to see why protein consumption is much higher than needed. When evaluating the protein content of animal-based foods, it is also important to evaluate what else these foods are (or are not) providing. Table 10-4 compares the nutritional content of animal- and plant-based foods. First, animal-based foods are more calorically dense than plant-based foods. Second, animal-based foods are very high in fat, especially saturated fat (while most plant-based foods are naturally low in fat). Third, animal-based foods are high in cholesterol whereas plant-based foods are naturally cholesterol free. Fourth, animal-based foods do not contain fiber, which has tremendous health benefit, while plant-based foods are naturally high in fiber. Fifth, animal-based foods are associated with a myriad of chronic diseases, such as cancer, cardiovascular disease, diabetes, autoimmune diseases, etc.

**Table 10-4 Nutritional content of plant- vs. animal-based foods**

|  | Plant-based foods | Animal-based foods |
| --- | --- | --- |
| **Caloric density** | Low | High |
| **Protein** | Easy to meet daily protein needs | Easy to consume more protein than needed daily |
| **Fat** | Low | Very high |
| **Cholesterol** | None | High |
| **Fiber** | High | Low |
| **Risk of chronic disease** | Lowered | Increased |

## Do I Need to Track My Protein Intake?

**No**. I have outlined the protein content of various foods for educational purposes. Most healthy adults consuming a wide variety of plant-based foods can easily meet their daily protein needs, and **do not** need to calculate the protein content of the foods they eat.

## What about Protein Supplements?

Protein or amino acid supplements in the form of powder or drinks are commonly sold and touted as providing essential nutrients or strengthening our muscles. There is no scientific evidence to support such claims.[1] A sensible diet can easily meet all of our daily protein needs. Furthermore, consuming excess proteins will not covert them to skeletal muscle or enhance strength. Our body will use the amino acids it needs to rebuild damaged or lost proteins, and the rest will be stored as fat.[1] The only way to increase muscle strength and bulk is through regular physical exercise.

It is important to note that dietary and herbal supplements are not regulated by the FDA in the same manner as prescription and over-the-counter medications. In 1994, Congress passed a bill, which was later signed into law, called the Dietary Supplement Health and Education Act (DSHEA). It defined dietary supplements as a product containing any of the following: vitamin, mineral, amino acid, herb, botanical, concentrate, metabolite, constituent, or extract.[4] DSHEA placed dietary supplements in a different category than medications, with the following rules applicable to supplements:[4]

- Unlike medications, manufacturers are not required to prove safety or efficacy of a supplement prior to marketing or selling it.
- Unlike medications, manufacturers are not required to report post-marketing adverse events to the FDA.
- In case of an adverse outcome, the burden of proof falls upon the FDA to prove that supplements are harmful, rather that the manufacturer to prove that they are safe.
- Supplement labels are required to state: "this product in not intended to diagnose, treat, cure, or prevent any disease." However, supplement labels can make health claims such as "for healthy bones, mood, and immune functions."

Supplements can and do lead to harm. Large quantities of amino acids can lead to diarrhea.[1] Excess consumption of one amino acid can interfere with absorption and transport of other amino acids and therefore lead to deficiency of other amino acids.[1] Supplements of tryptophan, an amino acid, have caused a rare blood disorder known as eosinophilia-myalgia syndrome (EMS) in more than 1,500 people.

EMS causes severe muscle and joint pain and extremely high fever, and has resulted in more than three dozen deaths.[1]

## Reading Nutrition Labels

Almost all prepackaged foods have labels disclosing the protein content. Here are sample labels from packages of dry garbanzo beans and soy milk.

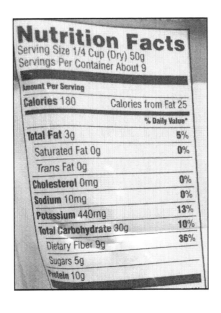

**Nutrition Facts**
Serving Size 1/4 Cup (Dry) 50g
Servings Per Container About 9

Amount Per Serving

Calories 180          Calories from Fat 25

% Daily Value*

| | |
|---|---|
| Total Fat 3g | 5% |
| Saturated Fat 0g | 0% |
| Trans Fat 0g | |
| Cholesterol 0mg | 0% |
| Sodium 10mg | 0% |
| Potassium 440mg | 13% |
| Total Carbohydrate 30g | 10% |
| Dietary Fiber 9g | 36% |
| Sugars 5g | |
| Protein 10g | |

**How to evaluate protein content of garbanzo beans**

- First thing we look at is the serving size.
- Each serving size is 1/4 cup of dry garbanzo beans.
- There are 180 calories per serving.
- There are 10g of protein per serving.
- 1g of protein = 4 calories.
- Thus, 40 out of the 180 calories per serving are from protein.
- 22% of the calories for each serving are from protein.

## How to evaluate protein content of soy milk

- First thing we look at is the serving size.
- Each serving size is 1 cup of soy milk.
- There are 80 calories per serving.
- There are 7g or protein per serving.
- 1g of protein = 4 calories.
- Thus, 28 out of the 80 calories per serving are from protein.
- 35% of the calories for each serving are from protein.

**Nutrition Facts**

Serving Size 1 Cup (240mL)
Servings Per Container 8

**Amount Per Serving**

| | |
|---|---|
| **Calories** 80 | Calories from Fat 35 |

| | % Daily Value* |
|---|---|
| **Total Fat** 4g | 6% |
| Saturated Fat 0.5g | 3% |
| Trans Fat 0g | |
| Polyunsaturated Fat 2.5g | |
| Monounsaturated Fat 1g | |
| **Cholesterol** 0mg | 0% |
| **Sodium** 70mg | 3% |
| **Potassium** 340mg | 10% |
| **Total Carbohydrate** 3g | 1% |
| Dietary Fiber 2g | 6% |
| Sugars 1g | |
| **Protein** 7g | 14% |

# Chapter 11
# What about All Those Vitamins & Minerals?

When it comes to vitamins and minerals, there are many opinions, questions, and a lot of confusion. You may be wondering if you are getting enough vitamins. Well-meaning friends and relatives may advise you to eat different foods in order to boost your intake of specific vitamins. The supplement aisle can seem overwhelming, as can the claims made by various supplement makers and food manufacturers. Which supplements do you need, and which ones are simply a waste of money and potentially dangerous? Let us review the answers in this chapter.

Before we move forward, it is important to remember that vitamin and mineral supplements are not regulated in the same manner by the FDA as medications. Supplement manufacturers do not have to prove that a product is safe or effective. In the event of an adverse outcome, the government has to prove cause and effect related to the supplement, and the manufacturer does not have to prove the safety of the supplement. Manufacturers are not required to report post-marketing adverse outcomes to the FDA.[1]

## What are Vitamins & Minerals

Vitamins and minerals are essential (with the exception of vitamin D) because our bodies cannot make them, and we must consume them in our diet. In terms of chemistry, vitamins are organic compounds, which means that they are complex molecules, whereas minerals are simple inorganic elements. Both vitamins and minerals are known as micronutrients because we only need to consume a small amount every day, i.e. a few micrograms to milligrams. Unlike carbohydrates, fats, and proteins, vitamins and minerals do not provide any kilocalories.

All minerals are water soluble, whereas vitamins can be water soluble or fat soluble. We generally need a small amount of water-soluble vitamins every day or every few days. Water-soluble vitamins are excreted by the kidneys. Fat-soluble vitamins are found in the fat or oil of foods and are stored in our body's fat. We need to consume fat-soluble vitamins every few weeks or months in order to avoid a deficiency.

### Table 11-1 Vitamins & minerals

| Minerals | Water-soluble vitamins | Fat-soluble vitamins |
|---|---|---|
| Calcium | Vitamin B1 (Thiamine) | Vitamin A |
| Sodium | Vitamin B2 (Riboflavin) | Vitamin D |
| Potassium | Vitamin B3 (Niacin) | Vitamin E |
| Iron | Biotin | Vitamin K |
| | Pantothenic Acid | |
| | Vitamin B6 | |
| | Folate | |
| | Vitamin B12 | |
| | Vitamin C | |

It is important to appreciate that both deficiency and toxicity of vitamins and minerals can lead to severe disease. Therefore, more is not always better. Toxicity is most often due to the use of supplements rather than dietary intake. Deficiencies of various vitamins and minerals are commonly seen in the developing world. In western countries, deficiencies are generally seen in special populations:[2]

- Alcoholics
- The elderly
- Dialysis patients
- Persons with certain gastrointestinal diseases such as celiac disease, Crohn's disease, pancreatic disease, or chronic diarrhea
- Individuals who have had gastric bypass surgery

If you have any of the medical conditions mentioned above, it is best to discuss your unique nutritional needs with your primary-care physician. Most healthy persons can meet their daily vitamins and mineral needs through their diets and do not need daily supplements. In the following sections, I will discuss those vitamins and minerals that commonly cause confusion, or for which deficiencies or excess are common.

- Folate
- Vitamin D
- Vitamin B12
- Calcium
- Iron
- Sodium
- Vitamin C

As we discuss various vitamins and minerals, it will be important to understand a few commonly used terms:

- **Recommended daily allowance (RDA)** is determined by the National Academy of Sciences, National Research Council, and the Institute of Medicine.[2] RDA is the amount of daily vitamin or mineral intake that will be sufficient to meet the needs of most healthy people. RDA for a specific nutrient may be different for different people based upon age, gender, pregnancy, and lactation.
- **Daily value (DV)** is established by the FDA to help consumers determine how much of a vitamin or nutrient is present in one serving size of food. There is a single DV for all persons over the age of four. Food labels do not list the absolute amount of a vitamin or nutrient present in a serving size. Rather, they show the percentage of DV per serving size.
- DV maybe equal to, less than, or greater than the RDA value for a specific nutrient.
- **Tolerable Upper Intake Level (UL)** is set for certain vitamins and minerals if excess consumption can lead to adverse consequences.[2] In order to prevent serious side effects and reactions, daily consumption should not exceed the UL.

## Folic Acid

You will often see the words "folate" and "folic acid" used interchangeably. Folate is the vitamin found naturally in foods such as green, leafy vegetables, fruits, cereals, grains, nuts, and meats.[2] Folic acid is the synthetic form of the vitamin that is found in supplements or fortified foods, such as flours, breads, rice, and cereals.[3] As discussed in Chapter 3, the federal government requires all products made from enriched grains to be fortified with folate.[4]

Folate deficiency can cause anemia and neural tube defects, a condition in which the spinal cord and brain do not form properly in the developing fetus. Most Americans obtain sufficient amounts of folate from their diet. Deficiency is usually seen in:[4]

- Alcoholics
- Patients with malabsorption due to celiac disease or inflammatory bowel disease
- Some women of child-bearing age

All adults need 400 µg of folate daily.[1,2] Adequate folic acid is particularly important for women of child-bearing age because folate deficiencies can lead to neural tube defects. Some women of child-bearing age do not consume enough folate. Since 50% of American pregnancies are unplanned, most experts recommend that all women of child-bearing age take a folate supplement of 400-800 µg every day.[2] The requirement is much higher for women planning a pregnancy who have a history of diabetes, neural tube defects, or take seizure medications.[3] If you are planning a pregnancy and have diabetes, or had a child with neural tube defects, or are taking seizure medication, you should discuss your folate requirements with your obstetrician.

Excessive folate intake can worsen B12 deficiency. This is most common with synthetic folic acid found in supplements and fortified foods, as it is better absorbed than folate found naturally in foods.

Therefore, the federal government has set a UL for synthetic folic acid taken in supplements or fortified foods.[4] The government has not set a UL for folate found naturally in food as adverse effects have not been reported from excessive food folate consumption.[4]

## Table 11-2 Folate

| Deficiency-related conditions | Sources | RDA[4] | DV[4] | UL[4] |
|---|---|---|---|---|
| Anemia<br><br>Neural tube defects | Natural sources: Green, leafy vegetables, fruits, cereals, grains, nuts, meats<br><br>Fortified foods: breads, rice, flour, cereals made from enriched grains. | All adults: 400 µg<br><br>Women of childbearing age 400-800 µg<br><br>Pregnancy 600 µg<br><br>Lactation 500 µg<br><br>Higher requirements for women planning a pregnancy who have diabetes, prior history of neural tube defects, or taking seizure medications. | Age 4 or greater: 400 µg | Age 19+ 1000 µg |

## Vitamin D

Vitamin D helps our body maintain calcium balance and bone health. Vitamin D deficiency is quite common and increases our risk of bone disease and fractures.

Our skin produces vitamin D in response to sun exposure. The amount produced varies with the amount of sun exposure, time of day, season, latitude, skin type, use of sun screens, genetic factors, and age.[5] Vitamin D is found naturally in very few foods, primarily fatty fish.[5] In the U.S., many foods are commonly fortified with vitamin D such as dairy milk, non-dairy milk, and cereals.[5] Vitamin D deficiency is quite common in the U.S. and around the world. Your physician can measure your vitamin D levels with a 'blood test in order to determine whether your levels are low or adequate. Daily requirements for vitamin D are usually expressed in micrograms ($\mu$g) or International Units (IU), where 1 IU is equivalent to 40 $\mu$g.

There are two types of vitamin D supplements available: vitamin D2 and vitamin D3. Some experts feel that vitamin D3 is more effective, while others feel that both are equally effective.[5,6] Supplements list the amount of vitamin D in terms of IU per tablet.

### Table 11-3 Vitamin D

| Deficiency-related conditions | Sources | RDA[5] | Daily Value[5] | UL[5] |
|---|---|---|---|---|
| Bone disease<br><br>Balance problems | Produced by skin in response to sun exposure<br><br>Fortified foods such as milks and cereals<br><br>Fatty fish | Ages 1-70: 600 IU<br><br>Age > 70: 800 IU | Age 4 or greater: 400 IU | Age 9 or greater: 4,000 IU |

Food items fortified with vitamin D list the amount of vitamin D in each serving as the percentage of daily value rather than the absolute amount of IU. To make matters more confusing, the daily value of of vitamin D is considered 400 IU based on older recommendations of 400 IU daily.[5] However, current daily recommendations are higher, as listed in Table 11-3.

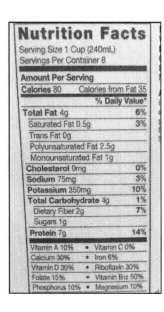

Reading nutrition label—soy milk

- Each serving size is 1 cup.
- Information about vitamins and minerals is listed towards the bottom of the label.
- Each serving size provides 30% of the daily value of vitamin D.
- The daily value is based on the old recommendation of 400 IU.
- 30% of 400 IU = 120 IU
- Each cup of soy milk provides vitamin D 120 IU.
- The current recommendation is for most adults under age 70 to consume vitamin D 600 IU daily.

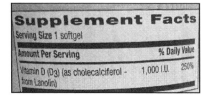

Vitamin D3 supplement label

- Each serving size is 1 tablet.
- Each tablet provides vitamin D3 1,000 IU
- The daily value is based on the old recommendation of 400 IU.
- Therefore each tablet provides 250% of the daily value.
- The current recommendation is for most adults under age 70 to consume vitamin D 600 IU daily.

## Vitamin B12

Vitamin B12 is important in the production of red blood cells, neurological function, and DNA synthesis. Microorganisms in the soil and intestines of animals produce vitamin B12.[7] In fact, microorganisms in our own intestines also synthesize vitamin B12, but we are not able to absorb it adequately.[7] When plants grow in healthy soil, they are able to absorb vitamin B12 produced by the microorganisms in the soil.[7] Most of the agriculture in the U.S. grows in soil that has been damaged from long-term use of unnatural pesticides, herbicides, and fertilizers. Therefore, our current plant products lack vitamin B12.[7]

Vitamin B12 is found naturally in almost all animal-based foods, such as meats, poultry, seafood, and dairy. For reasons mentioned above, plant foods generally do not contain vitamin B12 unless they are fortified. Cereals, nutritional yeast, plant-based milks, and meat analogues are commonly fortified with vitamin B12. Some plant foods, such as spirulina, sea vegetables, tempeh, and miso, may contain small amounts of B12 due to bacterial contamination.[9] However, the form and amount found in these products is not active or reliable.[9]

Deficiencies of vitamin B12 lead to anemia and neurological dysfunction, such as numbness, tingling, difficulty with balance, memory problems, or dementia. The element cobalt is found in vitamin B12 and therefore you will see the word "cobalamin" in the various forms and names of B12, such as cyanocobalamin and methylcobalamin.

## Table 11-4 Vitamin B12

| Deficiency-related conditions | Sources | RDA[8] | Daily Value[8] |
|---|---|---|---|
| Anemia | Supplements | Adults 2.4 µg/day | 6 µg/day |
| Neurological problems | Fortified foods such as cereals, plant-based milks, meat analogues, nutritional yeast | Pregnancy 2.8 µg/day | |
| | | Lactation 2.8 µg/day | |
| | Meats, poultry, dairy, seafood | | |

Most people in the U.S. obtain sufficient vitamin B12 from their diet. Deficiencies are most commonly seen in the following groups.

- Older adults, who may not produce enough stomach acid, which is necessary to absorb B12 found naturally in foods. However, they can still absorb B12 found in supplements and fortified foods. The Institute of Medicine, a U.S. government agency, recommends that all persons over age 50 consume B12 from a supplement or fortified foods.[8]
- Patients with pernicious anemia, who do not produce stomach acids or other factors that are necessary to absorb B12. They are often treated with intramuscular B12 or high doses of supplements.
- Individuals who have had gastrointestinal surgery, such as gastric bypass or removal of small intestine.
- Individuals with malabsorptive disorders, such as celiac disease and inflammatory bowel disease.
- Plant-based eaters, who should consume supplements or fortified foods.

Vitamin B12 supplements are sold individually or in multivitamin form. Many supplements contain doses of 100 µg, 500 µg, or 1000 µg, which is far more that the RDA of 2.4 µg. The higher doses are not harmful. For example, most healthy people only absorb about 10 µg of a 500 µg oral supplement.[8] The form of B12 in supplements is usually cyanocobalamin or methylcobalamin. Some experts advise cyanocobalamin while others feel that both are equally effective.[8,9]

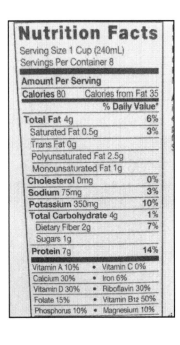

**Nutrition label - vitamin B12 in soy milk**

- Each serving size is 1 cup.
- Information about vitamins and minerals is listed towards the bottom of the label.
- Each serving size provides 50% of the daily value of vitamin B12.
- The daily value is 6 µg.
- 50% of 6 µg = 3 µg
- Each cup of soy milk provides 3 µg, which exceeds the RDA of 2.4 µg for most adults.

## Calcium

When most people think of calcium, they think of bones. While calcium is very important in bone and tooth health, it is also involved in the contraction and dilation of blood vessels, muscle contraction, nerve transmission, and helping our cellular parts communicate with each other. Less than 1% of our body's calcium is needed for these functions.[10] The remaining 99% is stored in our bones and teeth, where it helps support structure and function.[10]

Most of us have been taught that we need to consume dairy milk or yogurt in order to get enough calcium. However, as discussed in Chapter 2, dairy products have been associated with an increased incidence of Type 1 diabetes, multiple sclerosis, breast cancer, and prostate cancer. Additionally, countries with the highest incidence of dairy consumption have the highest fracture risk. Fortunately, calcium is abundant in many plant-based foods.[10,11] Most green, leafy vegetables and beans are rich in calcium. Spinach is an exception because it clings to calcium and prevents our bodies from absorbing it. Many foods are fortified with calcium, such as plant-based milks and juices. Some types of tofu, which are made using calcium, are also a good source.

While we need some calcium in our diets, just how much we need is unclear. Traditionally, the RDA for calcium has been 1,000mg for most adults and 1,200 mg for post-menopausal women.[10,12] Calcium supplements are widely available and have been touted for their positive impact on bone health. Many women have been taking calcium supplements in order to meet their daily requirement. However, calcium supplements are not benign medications and have been associated with kidney stones, constipation, and heart disease.

Recently, two important research studies have questioned the efficacy of dietary or supplemental calcium on bone health. Both studies, published in 2015 in the *British Medical Journal*, examined all studies involving calcium and bone health. A systemic review of the literature showed that calcium intake via the diet or supplements did

NOT reduce the incidence of osteoporotic fractures.[13] Another systemic review and meta-analysis of the literature showed that dietary and supplemental calcium increased bone mineral density by only about 0.6-1.8% after one year, and no further increases were seen thereafter.[14] Such an increase in bone density is minimal and highly unlikely to impact risk of fracture.[15] In light of these studies which were a review of all other studies on calcium and bone health, it is unclear what, if any, the RDA for calcium should be.

While we await further research to clarify the RDA for calcium, I advise taking the following steps to preserve bone health and minimize the risk of fractures.

- Exercise regularly, as both weight-bearing and strength-training exercises increase bone mineral density and decrease the risk for falls.[10-12]
- Stop smoking, as it increases calcium excretion and has been associated with low bone mineral density.[11,12]
- Limit alcohol to less than two drinks daily, as alcohol interferes with calcium absorption.[10,12]
- Limit caffeine consumption, as it increases calcium excretion. [10,11]
- Limit sodium intake, as sodium increases urinary calcium excretion.[10,11]
- Eat a whole-food, plant-based diet as it is associated with better bone health.[11]
- Obtain calcium from food sources, such as green, leafy vegetables, beans, and fortified plant-based milks, rather than dietary supplements.
- Consume adequate amounts of vitamin D, which is important in calcium balance and bone health.[10-12]

## Table 11-5 Calcium

| Functions | Sources | RDA | DV[10] | UL[10] |
|---|---|---|---|---|
| Bone health<br><br>Teeth health<br><br>Muscle contraction<br><br>Nerve transmission<br><br>Communication within cells<br><br>Contraction and dilation of blood vessels | Plant-based foods: Green, leafy vegetables, beans, tofu set in calcium, fortified plant-based milks, grains<br><br>Animal-based foods:<br>Dairy products | *Adults: 1,000 - 1,200 mg<br><br>*Merit of RDA unclear based upon recent research data | Age 4 or greater: 1000 mg | Age 19-50: 2,500 mg<br><br>Age 51+: 2,000 mg |

## Table 11-6 Calcium content of various plant-based foods

| | Calcium (mg) |
|---|---|
| Soymilk fortified 1 cup | 299 |
| Tofu firm calcium set 1/2 cup | 253 |
| Tofu soft calcium set 1/2 cup | 138 |
| Kale 1 cup raw | 100 |
| Collard greens boiled 1 cup | 266 |
| Bok choy 1 cup shredded | 74 |
| Broccoli raw 1/2 cup | 21 |
| Garbanzo beans cooked 1/2 cup | 40 |
| Navy beans 1/4 cup dry | 100 |

# Iron

Iron is a mineral that serves many important functions in our bodies: carrying oxygen in blood, storing oxygen in muscles, and helping various enzymes do their job. Iron deficiency can lead to developmental delay in children and anemia in persons of all ages.

Minimal amounts of iron are lost daily through sloughing of skin cells. Significant iron losses are due to blood loss, generally menstruation for women of childbearing age. However, for men and non-menstruating women, iron deficiency is usually due to blood loss from the urinary or gastrointestinal tract.

Iron is found in various animal- and plant-based foods such as red meats, poultry, fish, legumes, nuts, raisins, and dry peaches. Many cereals and breads are also fortified with iron.

Over-the-counter iron supplements are widely available. However, I recommend that iron supplements should only be consumed under the care of a physician for the following reasons:

- Iron deficiency may indicate blood loss due to a serious gastrointestinal or urinary tract disorder.
- The presence and severity of iron deficiency can be easily diagnosed with simple blood tests.
- Both iron deficiency and toxicity can lead to serious consequences.
- Some studies have suggested an increased risk of cancer and cardiovascular disease with increased iron stores.[16,17]

## Sodium

Unlike the other micronutrients we have reviewed, the problem with sodium is that most people consume **too much** rather than too little. Some sodium is found naturally in food. For example, small amounts of sodium are found naturally in vegetables, fruits, legumes, and whole grains. However, most of the sodium we consume is added to our food in the forms of additives, preservatives, and table salt. When most people think of sodium, they think of table salt. However, sodium and table salt (also known as sodium chloride) are not the same thing. Table salt is approximately 40% sodium and 60% chloride.[18] Besides table salt, sodium is found in many other food additives as shown in Table 11-7.[19]

**Table 11-7 Common sources of sodium in food other than table salt**

| Food additive | Example |
| --- | --- |
| Emulsifying agents | Sodium pyrophosphate |
| Buffering agents | Aluminum sodium sulfate |
| Anitcaking agents | Sodium aluminosilicate |
| Flavor-enhancing agents | Monosodium glutamate (MSG) |
| Leavening agents | Sodium bicarbonate (baking soda) |
| Dough-conditioning agents | Sodium stearoyl lactylate |
| Stabilizing agents | Disodium ethylenediaminetetraacetic acid (EDTA) |
| Neutralizing agents | Trisodium phosphate |
| Thickening agents | Sodium alginate |
| Moisture-retaining agents | Sodium hydrogen DL-malate |
| Texture-modifying agents | Sorbitol sodium |
| Bleaching agents | Sodium metabisulfite |

As we look at the myriad of additives that contain sodium, it is no surprise that most Americans consume too much sodium. Processed and restaurant foods are particularly high in sodium as they tend to use significant amounts of additives and table salt to reduce spoilage, prolong shelf life, improve texture, and enhance flavor. According to the CDC, over 75% of our sodium intake is from processed and restaurant foods. Figure 11-1 illustrates the sources of sodium in our foods.[20]

## Figure 11-1 Sources of dietary sodium

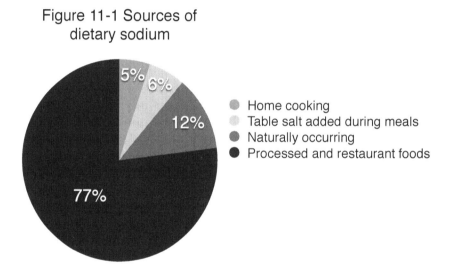

- Home cooking
- Table salt added during meals
- Naturally occurring
- Processed and restaurant foods

How much sodium do we need and how much are we actually consuming? According to the CDC, 90% of Americans eat too much sodium with the average American consuming 3,400mg of sodium daily.[21,22] Reducing the average sodium intake by 400mg could prevent up to 28,000 deaths per year, and save $7 billion in annual health care expenditures.[18] The recommended daily limits of sodium are far lower than 3,400mg and are outlined in Table 11-8.[23]

## Table 11-8 Daily limits on sodium

| Population | Daily limit |
|---|---|
| Age 2 or greater | 2,300 mg |
| Age 51 or greater | 1,500 mg |
| African Americans | |
| Patients with high blood pressure, chronic kidney disease, or diabetes | |
| Obese persons | |

What are the consequences of consuming too much sodium? High levels of sodium intake are associated with many serious conditions, as shown in Table 11-9.[23]

## Table 11-9 Health consequences of increased sodium intake

| Organ system | Conditions |
|---|---|
| Cardiovascular | Increased blood pressure |
| | Elevated heart rate |
| | Pathological thickening of heart muscle |
| Kidneys | Increased work load for kidneys |
| | Enhanced urinary calcium excretion thereby increasing risk of kidney stones and osteoporosis |
| Cancer | Increased risk of stomach cancer |
| Lungs | Asthma |
| Metabolic | Insulin resistance leading to increased blood sugar |

As we consume more sodium, our blood pressure increases, a phenomenon known as "salt sensitivity." Blood pressure of African Americans, older persons, obese individuals, patients with metabolic syndrome or chronic kidney disease are more sensitive to salt. Therefore, the daily limit on salt intake is lower for such persons.[23]

Given that the average American is consuming too much sodium and that excess sodium is harmful, how can we reduce our intake? Keeping in mind that most of our dietary sodium is from restaurant and processed foods, use the following tips to limit your sodium intake.

- Use the following as a visual cue: 1 teaspoon of salt = 2,300 mg of sodium.[18]
- Minimize your consumption of processed foods as they are very high in sodium. Fortunately, almost all processed foods you purchase in retail outlets have a nutrition label disclosing the amount of sodium in each serving. Look for foods that say low or no sodium on the label.
- Minimize consumption of restaurant meals that are not only high in sodium, but usually also high in sugar and fat. Nutritional information is not available for most restaurant meals, which makes it difficult to know the sodium content.
- Avoid keeping a salt shaker at the table. You are far less likely to add salt at the table if the shaker is not readily available.
- Foods do not have to taste salty in order to have high amounts of sodium. For example, some cheeses and breads can have high amounts of sodium even though they do not taste particularly salty.
- Use spices and herbs to season your food instead of salt. Try basil, cinnamon, chili, cilantro, mint, dill, etc.

## Vitamin C

Vitamin C, is also known as ascorbic acid. It is important for collagen synthesis, which is found in all connective tissue, such as skin, bone, muscle, tendons, ligaments, and teeth.[24] Vitamin C is also important in iron absorption, and has anti-oxidant properties.[24]

Most people think of oranges when they think of vitamin C. However, vitamin C is abundant in many other fruits and vegetables as well, such as red peppers, kiwi, and strawberries. Grains do not naturally contain vitamin C, and breakfast cereals that contain vitamin C are the result of fortification.[24]

### Table 11-10 Vitamin C

| Functions | Sources | RDA[24] | DV[24] | UL[24] |
|---|---|---|---|---|
| Collagen synthesis<br><br>Iron absorption<br><br>Anti-oxidant | Fruits: citrus, kiwi, strawberry, cantaloupe<br><br>Vegetables: tomatoes, potatoes, brussels sprouts, red sweet peppers, broccoli, cabbage, cauliflower, green peppers<br><br>Fortified cereals | Age 19 or greater<br>• Males 90mg/day<br>• Females 75mg/day<br><br>Pregnancy 85mg/day<br><br>Lactation 120mg/day<br><br>Smokers need an additional 35mg/day | Age 4 or greater: 60mg | Age 19 or greater: 2,000mg |

It is easy to meet our daily requirements for vitamin C through our diets. Table 11-11 shows the vitamin C content of commonly eaten fruits and vegetables. Most Americans consume enough vitamin C through their diet. Deficiencies are usually seen in the following individuals:[24]

- Smokers
- Infants fed evaporated or boiled cow's milk
- Patients with malabsorption or on hemodialysis
- Persons consuming a very restricted diet devoid of fruits and vegetables, such as the elderly or those who abuse alcohol or drugs.

**Table 11-11 Vitamin C content of various fruits and vegetables**

| Fruit | Vitamin C (mg) | Vegetable | Vitamin C (mg) |
|---|---|---|---|
| Medium orange | 70 | Sweet red pepper, 1/2 cup | 95 |
| Medium kiwi | 64 | Sweet green pepper, 1/2 cup | 60 |
| Strawberries, fresh, 1/2 cup sliced | 49 | Broccoli, raw, 1/2 cup | 39 |
| Grapefruit, 1/2 medium | 39 | Brussels sprouts, cooked, 1/2 cup | 48 |

Vitamin C supplements are widely available and advertised for their benefits in preventing cancer, cardiovascular disease, and the common cold. Research has not shown that vitamin C supplements reduce cardiovascular disease or cancer.[2,24] Many people take vitamin C supplements to prevent or treat the common cold. According to research data, supplements reduce the duration of a cold by 8%, and may reduce the incidence of the common cold by 50% in elite athletes who exercise vigorously under extreme conditions.[24,25]

The human body tightly controls how much vitamin C it needs, and excess amounts are not absorbed and excreted. Excess consumption through supplements can lead to diarrhea, nausea, abdominal cramps, and other gastrointestinal disturbances due to unabsorbed vitamin C.[24] Some research studies have also shown that vitamin C supplements can lead to kidney stones.[2,24]

Rather than using supplements, most of us should consume vitamin C naturally through fruits and vegetables as they provide many other nutrients and health benefits as well.

# Chapter 12
# Healthy Eating Habits and Our Food Environment

During my recent visit to New Delhi, I was very excited to reunite with my family. My cousins and I had grown up together, and I was thrilled to see them again after 14 years. They were very warm and welcoming, and invited us for lunch and dinner. During the meals, they kept lavishing us with home-cooked delicacies that had been prepared in our honor. Feeding us was their way of showing their love. As appreciative as I was of their sentiment and gesture, it was hard to keep eating. I was full but I didn't want to hurt their feelings. I found myself eating more than I normally would. In this chapter, I will explain how much of our eating behavior is determined by our environment.

Over the past few decades, the population of the United States has become heavier and unhealthier. Most of the weight gain is a byproduct of two developments: we are eating the wrong types of foods and we are eating too much of those foods. In the previous chapters, I have focused on what we should eat and which foods are healthy for us and which are not. While selecting the correct foods is paramount to our health, how we eat is also very important. Our eating habits and food environment play a big role in determining what we eat and how much we eat. In this chapter, we will explore the following aspects of our eating behavior.

- Why do we eat?
- When do we eat?
- How much do we eat?
- How does our food environment impact our eating behavior?
- How do our dining partners influence us?
- What do we do when we eat?

## Why Do We Eat?

There is only one reason we should eat: hunger. Sometimes, we are genuinely hungry and we eat to satisfy our hunger. Too often though, we eat for reasons other than hunger. These are some of the most common reasons why we eat:

- Stress
- Celebration
- Fatigue or insufficient sleep
- Boredom
- Social pressure

Some people eat less when they are stressed, while others may turn to food for comfort. Relationship conflicts, work stress, health problems, or financial hardship may trigger some people to eat even though they are not hungry. This type of eating is known as emotional eating.[1] Food provides comfort and a distraction from the stressful situation. If you find yourself eating more at stressful times, it may be beneficial to seek help from a behavioral professional who specializes in emotional eating, such as a licensed clinical social worker or a clinical psychologist.

Sometimes eating is triggered by positive emotions such as a birthday, job promotion, reaching an important milestone, vacation, or a holiday. Too often, celebrating is associated with consuming significant amounts of unhealthy foods. Common examples are Halloween, where children (and some adults) may eat quite a bit of candy in one day, or Thanksgiving, when most people eat a large amount of food in one meal. While it is important to celebrate the special moments in our life, we do not have to consume unhealthy foods or large amounts of food in order to do so. We could eat only as much as we need to satisfy our hunger at a family celebration, and save the rest for a later meal.

People often reach for food when they are tired of working or studying, or have had insufficient sleep. Food distracts us from our fatigue and gives us a sudden burst of energy. However, the energy and distraction are short lived, and we soon feel tired again. Rather than turning to food, we can try other strategies to alleviate our fatigue. If we are tired from a desk job, try a little exercise or fresh air. If we are tired from physical work, try sitting or laying down for a while. Research has shown that people who sleep less, eat more on the following day. If you are sleep deprived, try a short nap.

Sometimes we eat because we are bored, food is available, and because we can eat it. This type of mindless eating can lead to a significant amount of caloric intake. Instead of reaching for food, we can try exercising, reading, or engaging in a hobby.

Often we eat because our family members or hosts have prepared a special meal for us and we want to show our appreciation by eating it. Growing up in India, I often felt the pressure to eat meals that my relatives had worked hard to prepare. Sometimes we eat just because everyone around us is eating and we want to blend in. For example, noshing at an office party. In each of these situations, the smarter approach is to converse and engage socially with others while delaying eating until hungry.

## When Do We Eat?

Many people eat three major meals a day: breakfast, lunch, and dinner. The problem with this approach is that we are very likely to become hungry in between the meals and then overeat during each meal. In order to understand why, it is important to appreciate our hunger and satiety scales, as illustrated in Table 12-1. Our hunger level can range from feeling content to starving. Similarly, our satiety level can range from feeling content to painfully full.

## Table 12-1 Hunger and satiety

| Hunger and satiety level | Sensation |
| --- | --- |
| Starving | All you can think about is food and at this point you will most likely overeat. |
| Hungry | Food is very much on your mind. If you do not eat immediately, you are very likely to overeat. |
| Starting to feel hungry | You are starting to think about food and feel hungry. This is the time to arrange for your next meal and plan to eat soon. |
| Content | This is where you want to be. Neither hungry nor full. Just comfortable. |
| Full | Your stomach feels a little fuller than it should and you have likely eaten more than you should. |
| Stuffed | Your stomach is really full and you are starting to feel uncomfortable. |
| Painfully full | Your stomach is extremely full and you are in pain. It is hard to function. |

Ideally, we want to stay in the green zone as much as possible. We want to feel content, neither hungry not full. We should eat soon after we start to feel hungry. If we do not do so, our feelings of hunger will only grow stronger. If we let ourselves get too hungry, we are very likely to overeat and binge rather than selecting healthy foods and eating sensible portion sizes. Similarly, while we are eating, we should stop eating once we no longer feel hungry, and before we start to feel full. If we do not stop as soon we no longer feel hungry, we are likely to overeat and then feel full. Eventually, we will feel stuffed and worse yet, be in pain. How can we stay in the green zone? By eating six moderate-sized meals a day rather than three large meals. Table 12-2 illustrates six small meals in a typical day.

### Table 12-2 Six small daily meals

| Meal | Examples |
| --- | --- |
| **Breakfast** | Oatmeal with soy milk and fresh fruits |
| **Mid-morning snack** | Apple slices with peanut butter |
| **Lunch** | Whole-grain sandwich with hummus, veggies, and sprouts |
| **Mid-afternoon snack** | Toast with avocado and tomatoes |
| **Dinner** | Veggies Tacos |
| **Late evening snack** | Toast with jam or fresh fruit |

Will eating more meals daily lead to weight gain? No. We are converting three large meals to six smaller meals daily. While we are eating more often, we are eating less at each meal, and our overall caloric intake is decreasing. Furthermore, by feeling content most of the day, you are more likely to make sensible food choices. Whereas when we are very hungry or starving, we are much more likely to reach for whatever is available and overeat.

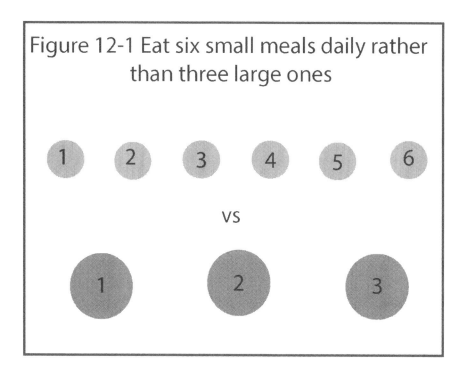

Figure 12-1 Eat six small meals daily rather than three large ones

Many people skip breakfast either because they are rushing or because they are simply not hungry. Breakfast is just as important as other meals. Eating soon after we wake up sends a signal to our bodies that it is time to go and expend some energy. If you are not hungry in the mornings, it may be because you ate a big meal shortly before going to bed.

I would like to make a special note about the late evening snack. While it is not advisable to eat a large meal before going to bed, it is also not a good idea to go to bed hungry. It can be difficult to sleep with a full or hungry stomach. Try to opt for a simple and light late-evening snack, such as a slice of whole grain bread or fruit.

## How Much Do We Eat?

Some of the biggest drivers of our obesity epidemic have been our increasing portion sizes. Over the past few decades, portion sizes of food and drinks at almost all restaurants have increased significantly. Even the sizes of coffee, soft drinks, and movie popcorn have increased. Tables 12-3[2] and 12-4[3] outline how much the portions of commonly-eaten foods have increased with time.

As we see in Tables 12-3 and 12-4, portion sizes have increased drastically and most meals provide over twice the calories that they once did. Meals at most restaurants are now family sized rather than individual sized. When we are served larger meals, we tend to eat more. While larger-sized meals are often marketed as better value for our money, we the consumer do not benefit overall from them. We either end up eating more than we need, gaining weight and jeopardizing our health, or we throw out the excess food.

Larger portion sizes at a single restaurant meal do not simply impact how much we eat at that specific meal. They also have long-lasting impact on our sense of satiety and our portion sizes in subsequent meals. Large portion sizes leave us feeling full and stuffed, rather than content. With time, we become accustomed to this level of fullness after each meal, and keep eating until we reach it. Thus we develop a pattern of eating a larger amount of food each time we eat.

## Table 12-3 Increasing portion sizes over the past 20 years

| Food item | Average serving size and calories 20 years ago | Serving size and calories today | Net increase in calories |
|---|---|---|---|
| Bagel | 3" diameter<br><br>140 calories | 6" diameter<br><br>350 calories | 240 |
| Spaghetti and meatballs | 1 cup spaghetti with sauce and 3 small meatballs<br><br>500 calories | 2 cup spaghetti with sauce and 3 large meatballs<br><br>1025 calories | 525 |
| Soda | 6.5 oz<br><br>85 calories | 20 oz<br><br>250 calories | 165 |
| Coffee | 8 oz with whole milk and sugar<br><br>45 calories | 16 oz with steamed whole milk and mocha syrup<br><br>350 callers | 305 |
| Turkey sandwich | 320 calories | 820 calories | 500 |
| Blueberry muffin | 1.5 oz<br><br>210 calories | 4 oz<br><br>500 calories | 290 |
| Chicken caesar salad | 1.5 cups<br><br>390 calories | 3.5 cups<br><br>790 calories | 400 |
| Movie popcorn | 5 cups<br><br>270 calories | 11 cups<br><br>630 calories | 360 |
| Cheesecake | 3 oz<br><br>260 calories | 7 oz<br><br>640 calories | 380 |
| Chocolate chip cookie | 1.5 inch diameter<br><br>55 calories | 3.5 inch diameter<br><br>275 calories | 220 |
| Chicken stir fry | 2 cups<br><br>534 calories | 4.5 cups<br><br>865 calories | 430 |

## Table 12-4 Super-sizing of various foods over the years

| Food item | Then | Now |
|-----------|------|-----|
| **Hershey Milk Chocolate Bar** | 1908: 0.6 oz | 2004: 1.6 oz, 2.6 oz, 4 oz, 7 oz, 8oz |
| **McDonald's French Fries**[3,4] | 1955: McDonald's offers fries in one size only: 2.4 oz | 2015: McDonald's fries come in 4 sizes<br><br>kids 1.3 oz (110 calories)<br>small 2.6 oz (230 calories)<br>medium 3.9 oz (340 calories)<br>large 5.9 oz (510 calories) |
| **McDonald's Hamburger**[3,5,6] | 1955: first hamburger has 1.6 oz precooked beef | 2015: McDonald's hamburger comes in many sizes<br><br>Quarter Pounder cheese burger contains 4.25 oz. of precooked beef and provides 540 calories<br><br>Double Quarter Pounder cheeseburger contains 8.5 oz. of precooked beef and provides 780 calories |
| **McDonald's soda**[3,7] | 1955: only one size available, 7 oz | 2015: McDonald's now offers sodas in 4 sizes<br><br>X-small 12 oz<br>Small 16 oz<br>Medium 21 oz<br>Large 30 oz |
| **Pizza Hut pizza**[3,8] | 1975: Pizza Hut offers one size, 10" diameter | 2015: Pizza hut offers 3 sizes<br><br>Personal pan 6" diameter<br>Medium 12" diameter<br>Large 14" diameter |

## How Does Our Food Environment Impact Our Eating Behavior?

Dr. Brian Wansink, Ph.D., is director of Cornell University's Food and Brand Lab, and a leading expert in eating behavior.[9] His research has shown that our food environment has a tremendous impact on what we eat and how much we eat. The manner in which our food is served, the eating utensils we use, and the arrangement of food around us can impact the choices we make.

For example, the kind of food that is most readily visible around our kitchen is the food we are most likely to eat. Research has shown that we are much more likely to eat fruits if they are readily visible around the kitchen or dining room area. Similarly, we are much more likely to eat candies if there is a "candy jar" in plain sight. When it comes to unhealthy foods, the old adage "out of sight, out mind," is spot on.

When you eat at home, do you keep the serving platters on the table or away from the table? When the serving platters are located on the table, we are much more likely to get second or third servings. However, if we have to get up and walk to get more food, we are much less likely to reach for seconds or thirds. When food is served from the stove or counter, people eat 19% less food than when food is served straight off the table.[9]

The sizes of the serving platters are also important. When food is served from smaller platters with smaller utensils, we tend to take less and eat less.[9] The same food served from larger platters or with large utensils, will drive us to take more and eat more.

Plate size and color play a critical role in how much we eat. As shown in Table 12-5, the average plate size has increased over time. Figure 12-2 illustrates how the same amount of food appears to be less in a larger plate, and therefore we eat more of it.[9] The color of our plates is also important. When the colors of our food and plate or bowl are the same, we serve ourselves 18% more food.[9]

### Table 12-5 Increasing plate size over the years

| Year | Average plate size[10] |
|------|------------------------|
| 1900 | 9 inches |
| 1950 | 10 inches |
| 2010 | 12 inches |

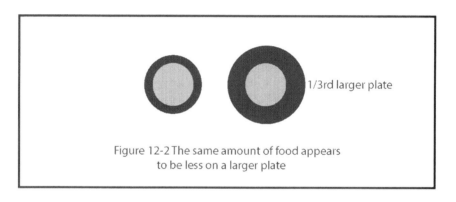

1/3rd larger plate

Figure 12-2 The same amount of food appears
to be less on a larger plate

The sizes and shapes of our glasses affect how much we drink. We judge the volume of our drinks by their height rather than their width. Let us assume that we pour the same amount of fluid in two cups, one of which is tall and thin, while the other is short and wide. The tall and thin cup will appear to have more volume because the height of the beverage is higher.[9] Over the years, the size of the average cup has increased. I grew up in India, drinking from cups which were 5-6 ounces in volume. Currently, most coffee cups and tumblers are significantly large often well over 12 ounces. Just as with plates, larger cups encourage us to drink more volume.

All-you-can-eat buffets are quite popular and may seem like a good bargain. However, we are much more likely to overeat in such a setting in order to get our money's worth. People who sit closer to the buffet or who face the buffet are much more likely to eat more than those whose backs are to the buffet or are seated far away.[9] Larger plates at a buffet induce us to eat more.[9] People who survey all of the food choices prior to serving themselves make healthier choices than people who serve the food without surveying the options.[9]

## How Do Our Dining Partners Influence Us?

Men generally eat faster than women and eat a larger volume than women.[9] This can lead to a negative impact on both partners. My husband is bigger than me and tends to eat very fast. When I dine with him, I often find myself trying to match his portion size and eating speed. This is not a conscious effort on my part—it is human nature to subconsciously imitate one another. It is much healthier for us to chew slowly and take our time eating. Since men eat quickly, after they are done eating, they often continue to eat a second or third portion in order to accompany their slower dining partners.[9]

We are also influenced by what others around us are eating. For example, it is much harder to resist ice cream if everyone around us is eating it. On the other hand, we are much more likely to resist dessert if no one else is having any.

## What Do We Do When We Eat?

What do you like to do while you eat? Do you engage in any of the following activities while eating?

- Watch TV
- Use your phone, tablet or laptop
- Read
- Listen to the radio
- Drive
- Walk

If you do, then you are not alone. Many people watch TV, read, or use an electronic device while eating. Some drive or walk while snacking. The problem is that all of these tasks distract us, and then we are the very likely to miss the signal from our brain telling us that we are full, resulting in overeating.[9] So what should we do when we eat? First, we should sit comfortably while we eat. If we are with others, simple conversation will slow down our eating. When dining alone, it is healthier to simply eat without distraction. While this may sound boring, it works remarkably well in helping us judge when we are satisfied. Eating then becomes a meditative experience where we enjoy the food, and become well attuned to our satiety signals. After moving to the U.S., I really enjoyed eating while watching TV, and this became my way of eating and relaxing. Years later, I decided to break my unhealthy habit. The first time I tried eating alone without TV, I was concerned that I would feel really bored and not enjoy my meal. However, I was surprised at how much less I ate, and that I did not miss the distraction as much as I thought I would.

In the American culture, television and movies are often associated with eating. For example, pizza and beer during a football game, or popcorn and soda at a movie theater. Although it seems tempting to eat while being entertained, this often leads to mindless overeating. It is important to dissociate our need for food from our need for entertainment. Eat before or after the movie, just not while watching it!

### Table 12-5 Summary of healthy food environment

| | Healthy | Avoid |
|---|---|---|
| **Food arrangement and storage** | Make fruits readily visible in the kitchen and refrigerator | Keeping non-nutritious foods in plain sight such as candies, chips, chocolates, cookies, etc. |
| **Plates, cups and utensils** | Use salad size plates rather than dinner size plates | Dinner-size plates |
| | Use plates with colors that contrast with the food | Plates that have the same color as the food |
| | Use smaller cups, 6-8 oz | Cups or glasses larger than 8oz |
| | Use smaller utensils | Large forks, knives, or spoons |
| **Serving food** | Serve food from small platters | Serving food from large platters |
| | Serving food away from the table | Serving food at the table |
| **All-you-can-eat buffet (best to avoid)** | Sit far from the buffet | Sitting close to buffet |
| | Do not face the buffet | Facing the buffet while seated |
| | Survey all of the food options, before selecting any | Selecting items without surveying all of them |
| | Avoid returning for seconds | Going for seconds or thirds |
| | Choose smaller plates | Choosing large plates |
| **Dining partner** | Eating slowly and only as much as you need | Eating fast to match your partner's speed |
| | | Eating more to match your partner's volume |
| **Distractions** | Avoid all distractions such as TV, electronic devices, reading, listening to radio | Eating while watching TV, speaking on phone, using any type of electronic device, radio, walking, driving. |
| | Avoid eating while walking or driving | |
| | Eat while seated comfortably | |

## Table 12-6 Summary of healthy eating habits

|  | Healthy | Avoid |
|---|---|---|
| **Reason for eating** | Hunger | Stress, celebration, boredom, fatigue, social pressure |
| **Timing of meals** | Eat 6 small meals daily | A few large meals daily |
| **Satiety** | Eat soon after you start to feel hungry<br><br>Eat until you are content: neither hungry not full | Letting yourself get too hungry or too full |

# Chapter 13
# **Dessert - How Sweet Is Too Sweet?**

**I** love to travel with my family and explore different countries and sights. As a physician with a special interest in nutrition, I really enjoy studying other cultures, and their cuisines and lifestyles. A few years ago, my family and I visited Hong Kong. We were enjoying afternoon tea while overlooking beautiful Victoria Harbor. As I nibbled on the cookies on my plate, I noticed that the cookies were not nearly as sweet as the ones we get in the U.S. In fact, they were barely sweet by American standards. A thought started to form in my mind: are our desserts too sweet?

After returning home, I started my own experimentation with desserts. My daughter loves to bake and bakes most of our desserts for us. Each time she found a recipe to try, we cut the sugar content by 30-50%. I was curious if using less sugar than the recipe suggested would diminish the taste. Surprisingly, it did not. We all enjoyed the desserts just as much!

Over time, our taste buds became accustomed to desserts that were less sweet than commercially-prepared ones. Now, when we do have store-bought ice cream or cookies, we find them to be too sweet. While desserts are not essential from a nutrition standpoint, desserts are an important part of most cultures and daily life. A simple way to make our desserts more nutritious is to simply minimize how much sweeteners we add to them. You can do this easily at home by cutting the amount of added sweeteners in most recipes by 30-50%. When dining in restaurants, it is not possible to reduce the amount of sweeteners used to prepare desserts. However, we can minimize how many other sweet treats we add to our desserts such as sprinkles, caramel, chocolate syrup, whipped cream, etc. Another option is to simply reduce the amount of dessert we consume. Most restaurants have increased their dessert portions significantly, and a single dessert can easily satisfy the sweet tooth of two to four persons. If you are dining alone, order kids'-sized desserts. For example, ordering a kids'-size scoop of ice cream in a cup, and avoiding the cone, syrups, and sweet toppings.

## Chocolate

Many people enjoy chocolate. You may have heard through media reports that dark chocolate is good for us. What is dark chocolate? How is it different from milk or white chocolate?

Chocolate is made from cocoa beans. The health benefits of chocolate come from flavanols, which are found in cocoa beans. Flavanols have several health benefits:[1]

- They include antioxidants, which help our bodies repair damage.
- They reduce blood pressure.
- They improve blood flow to the brain and heart.
- They make our blood less likely to clot.

Flavanols are also found in other plant-based foods, such as cranberries, apples, peanuts, onions, tea, and red wine. As cocoa beans are processed into chocolate, many of the flavanols are lost.[1]

Cocoa beans contain two main ingredients: cocoa butter and cocoa. The amount of cocoa in a chocolate bar determines whether it is dark, milk, or white. Dark chocolate is made from cocoa, cocoa butter, sugar, and vanilla. Dark chocolates usually do not contain any milk powder, but some may. Milk chocolate is also made from cocoa, cocoa butter, sugar, and flavor. Unlike most dark chocolates, milk powder is added to milk chocolates. Compared to dark chocolates, milk chocolates contain less cocoa and more sugar. Therefore, milk chocolates are sweeter and less bitter than dark chocolates.

White chocolates do not contain any cocoa. They are made from cocoa butter, milk, sugar, and flavor. Therefore, white chocolate is much sweeter than dark or milk chocolate.

You may have noticed "% cacao" or "% cocoa" on chocolate labels. The percentage refers to percentage of total weight, which is comprised of cocoa and cocoa butter. As the percentage of cacao increases, the  amount of added sugar decreases, and the sweetness decreases. The percentage content of cocoa in various chocolates is outlined in Table 13-1.

### Table 13-1 Types of chocolates

| Chocolate | Percentage cacao by weight | Sweetness and added sugar | Bitterness |
|---|---|---|---|
| Milk | At least 10% | Sweetest | Not bitter |
| Semi-sweet and bitter sweet | At least 35% | Moderately sweet | Mild to moderately bitter |
| Dark | 50-90% | Mildly sweet | Mild to moderately bitter |
| 100% baking chocolate or 100% cocoa powder | 100% | Not sweet at all | Very bitter |

Dark chocolate contains more flavanols than milk or white chocolate. It is also lower in sugar and does not contain milk. Therefore, dark chocolates are healthier for us than milk or white chocolate. If you are accustomed to eating milk chocolates, you may find dark chocolates a little bitter initially. However, if you consistently eat dark instead of milk chocolate, your palate will adjust to a lower level of sweetness. You will then enjoy the less sweet taste of dark chocolate and find milk chocolate to be too sweet.

Cocoa powder is 100% cacao. If you are using cocoa powder, avoid Dutch processed ones because some of the flavanols are lost during the processing.[1] In Dutch processing, the natural acidity of the cocoa powder is reduced by adding an alkalizing agent.

## Tips for Eating Desserts

Desserts are all around us and a part of most cultures. Naturally, we all crave desserts as we watch others eat them. The problem with most desserts is that they are very calorically dense, as they are often loaded with sugar and fat. Additionally, most restaurants now serve family-sized rather than individual-sized desserts. The key with desserts is to eat them in moderation and minimize the fat and sugar content to the extent possible. Here are some tips that may help you.

- Whenever possible, make your own desserts at home. This way you can minimize how much sugar or other sweeteners you add.
- Whenever you reach for chocolate, opt for darker varieties over milk or white.
- Although dark chocolates are healthier than lighter varieties, they are still high in calories and fat. Try to limit the serving size of dark chocolate to 0.5 oz. each time and pair it with fresh fruits, such as strawberries or raspberries.

- Use very small plates and utensils to eat desserts. This way you will eat less.
- Many restaurant desserts are now large enough for 2-4 persons to share. Share desserts with family and friends in restaurants rather than getting your own. You will save money and calories.
- If you are dining alone, pack a portion of the serving to take home with you for a later time.
- Order kids'-sized ice cream in a cup, and avoid the cone and other toppings.

# Chapter 14
# Beware of Liquid Calories

At the end of each high school day, I was famished! One day, on the way home on the school bus, one of my friends was eating a Snickers candy bar with Coca-cola. I was starving and this combination looked delicious. The sweet, nutty, salty taste of the candy bar coupled perfectly with the sweet, carbonated, cool beverage. Soon, these became my favorite after-school snacks. Little did I realize that I was consuming nearly 500 empty calories on a daily basis.

## Calories in Common Beverages

Drinking sweetened or alcoholic beverages with meals and snacks has become common practice in the U.S. and many other countries. Furthermore, as we explored in Chapter 11, the serving sizes of most beverages have doubled or even tripled over the years. The majority of sit-down restaurants serve beverages prior to serving meals. When we are hungry, it is easy for us to fill up with large amounts of liquid calories while waiting for our food. It is important to note that most of these drinks are loaded with empty calories and lack nutritional value. The result is that many people unknowingly ingest a large number of calories every day from alcoholic and non-alcoholic drinks. Table 14-1 outlines the caloric content of common beverages.

### Table 14-1 Caloric content of common beverages

| Drink | Calories |
|-------|----------|
| Coca-Cola 12 oz. can[1] | 140 |
| Coca-Cola 16 oz. bottle[1] | 190 |
| Minutemaid Orange juice 8 oz.[1] | 110 |
| Minutemaid Apple juice 15.2 oz.[1] | 210 |
| Starbucks kids 8 oz. hot chocolate with 2% milk and whip cream[2] | 230 |
| Starbucks caffe latte tall (12 oz.) with whole milk without sugar[2] | 180 |
| Starbucks Mocha Frappuccino grande (16 oz.) with whole milk and whip cream[2] | 410 |
| Red wine 5 oz.[3] | 125 |
| White wine 6 oz.[3] | 121 |
| Beer 12 oz.[3] | 153 |

## How Many Calories Do We Consume from Drinks Every Day?

Table 14-2 provides an illustration of how many liquid calories a typical American may ingest in a given day, as well as healthier alternatives. As we see in Table 14-2, the average American can easily consume **over 1000 calories daily from beverages that have little or no nutritional value**. Even these numbers may underestimate the true intake of liquid calories. For example, most restaurants' serving size of orange juice is closer to 12 or 16 oz. rather than the 8 oz. used in Table 14-2. Many restaurants continue to refill large soda glasses, free of charge, while consumers are dining. Rather than drinking orange juice, we are far better off eating an orange, as the actual fruit provides fiber and other nutrients that are lost during juicing at a lower caloric cost. A whole milk espresso drink with whip cream is loaded with calories, saturated fat, and cholesterol. Instead opt for a soy latte, as soy milk is naturally low in saturated fat and cholesterol free.

Table 14-2  Illustration of liquid calorie consumption in a given day

| Meal | Beverage | Calories | Healthier option | Calories |
|------|----------|----------|------------------|----------|
| **Breakfast** | Orange juice 8 oz. | 110 | Orange[3] | 62 |
| **Lunch** | Coca-cola 16 oz | 190 | Water | 0 |
| **Afternoon coffee[2]** | Starbucks Grande (16 oz) Mocha Frappauccino with whole milk and whip cream | 410 | Starbucks Short (8 oz.) latte with soy milk | 90 |
| **Dinner[3]** | 2 Beers, 12 oz each | 306 | Red wine 5 oz. | 125 |
| **Total daily beverage calories** | | **1016** | | **277** |

## Are Artificially Sweetened Drinks Healthy?

There are many types of alternative sweeteners available, and Table 14-3 outlines the ones commonly used in the U.S. Most alternative sweeteners are calorie free with the following exceptions:

- Aspartame provides 4 kcal/g just as sugar does. However, aspartame is 200 times sweeter than sugar, and therefore very little is used, and the caloric count is negligible.
- Sugar alcohols provide 1.6-2.6 kcal/g compared to 4 kcal/g with sugar. However, sugar alcohols are notorious for causing gastrointestinal symptoms such as intestinal gas, abdominal bloating, and diarrhea.

It is tempting to think that alternatively sweetened drinks are healthier for us because they offer the sweet taste without the calories. However, alternative sweeteners are not healthy for the following reasons.

- As we see in Table 14-3, most alternative sweeteners are 200-600 times sweeter than sugar. Such a high level of sweetness reinforces our craving for sweetness and we tend to keep seeking out sweeter foods at the cost of other unsweetened nutritious foods.
- Alternatively-sweetened beverages can lead to overeating in the following manner: zero-calorie beverages confer a false sense of security that they are healthy, and thereby people may drink large volumes of them. Even though we may not ingest any calories from large volumes of these beverages, our stomach becomes accustomed to the fullness imparted by them. With subsequent meals, we tend to eat until we reach the same level of fullness rather than stopping when we are no longer hungry.

## Table 14-3 Alternative sweeteners

| Alternative sweetener | Trade name | Sweetness relative to sugar | Calories per gram | Well known side effects |
|---|---|---|---|---|
| **Aspartame** | NutraSweet, Equal, Canderel | 200x | 4 | |
| **Saccharin** | Sweet'N Low | 450x | 0 | |
| **Sucralose** | Splenda | 600x | 0 | |
| **Stevia** | Sweetleaf, Purevia, Truvia, Honey Leaf | 300x | 0 | |
| **Sugar alcohols (Isomalt, Lactitol, Maltitol, Mannitol, Sorbitol, Xylitol)** | | 0.4 - 1.0x | 1.6 - 2.6 | Intestinal gas, abdominal discomfort, diarrhea |

If you prefer tea or coffee with a sweet taste (as I do), it is best to add a small amount of sugar or another natural sweetener rather than an alternative sweetener. It is best to avoid alternative sweeteners for the reasons stated above. As I mentioned in Chapter 8, there are many available sweeteners such as table sugar, brown sugar, agave, honey, etc. No one sweetener is better than another, and I recommend selecting one based upon taste and convenience.

## Helpful Tips with Beverages

- Always drink water with every meal, as it is the best way to quench our thirst.
- Eat fresh fruits rather than drinking fruit juices.
- Avoid all alternative sweeteners as they encourage overeating and sweet cravings.
- Women should limit their alcoholic beverages to one serving, and men should limit them to no more than two.
- As a general rule, it is best to avoid all sodas. However, if you do crave them sometimes, limit your intake to 5-6 oz.
- When drinking coffee or tea, limit your serving size to 5-8 oz. rather than the 12, 16, or 20 oz. which have become standard at most coffee shops.
- If you prefer to sweeten your tea or coffee, add a small amount of a natural rather than alternative sweetener.

# Chapter 15
# Why Exercise Alone Is Not Enough

During medical school, one of my friends was an avid runner who exercised daily. She encouraged me to jog, and I loved it! Following her example, I started to work out on a daily basis. Within a few months, I had lost a great deal of weight and was very happy with the results. I thought that I could eat anything I wanted as long I exercised it off. However, I gradually regained the weight despite exercising regularly. Even though I was disappointed with the weight gain, I continued to exercise daily because it made me feel good—I felt energized and empowered.

In this chapter, I will explain why exercise alone isn't enough to lead to long-term weight loss. Exercise has many health benefits. However, exercise is not a substitute for healthy nutrition and cannot compensate for poor eating habits.

Regular physical exercise is important for every body. The WHO and the 2008 Physical Activity Guidelines for Americans advise all adults to engage in at least 150 minutes of moderate intensity aerobic exercises or 75 minutes of vigorous intensity aerobic exercises every week.[1] The American Heart Association and the American College of Sports Medicine have similar recommendations:[1]

- Moderate intensity exercises for at least 30 minutes for a minimum of five days a week.
- Or strenuous exercise for at least 20 minutes for a minimum of three days a week.

Regular physical exercise has a myriad of health benefits, which are outlined in Table 15-1. Despite the well-known benefits of exercise, less than 40% of adults meet the recommended daily amounts of exercise.[2] Furthermore, only 13 to 34% of patients report exercise advice from their primary care physicians.[1]

#### Table 15-1 Health benefits of regular physical exercise

| Organ System | Benefits from exercise[1] |
| --- | --- |
| Overall | Reduce mortality |
| | Help with weight management |
| Cardiovascular | Reduce the risk of hypertension |
| | Reduce blood pressure in persons with hypertension |
| | Reduce the risk of dying from heart disease |
| | Reduce the risk of stroke |
| Cancer | Reduce the risk of colon cancer |
| Endocrine | Reduce the risk of diabetes |
| Psychological | Reduces anxiety and depression |
| | Promote sense of well being |
| Musculoskeletal | Increase bone, joint and muscle strength |
| | Improve balance and strength in elderly persons |

As Table 15-1 outlines, regular physical exercise has tremendous health benefits, and almost all adults should engage in regular physical exercise. However, regular exercise does not replace healthy nutrition and cannot overcome a poor diet for several reasons.

First, animal-based foods are associated with excess weight and most chronic illnesses, such as cardiovascular disease, cancer, and auto-immune illnesses. On the other hand, a whole-food, plant-based diet reduces the risk of obesity and most chronic diseases, and can even reverse them. Therefore, even with regular exercise, it is still important to eat a whole-food, plant-based diet.

Second, exercise alone is not an effective way to lose or maintain weight. We can easily consume a large number of calories within a few minutes, while it takes hours of exercise to burn off the same calories. Table 15-2 lists the calories consumed during common forms of exercises, and Table 15-3 lists the caloric content of commonly consumed foods. For example, a person can eat two slices of pepperoni pizza, totaling 850 calories, within 10 minutes. However, even after biking for 85 minutes, a 160 pound person would burn 500 calories, far less than those found in the pizza slices.

Third, people can actually gain weight with exercise. Obviously, this is not a problem if the weight gain is solely due to an increase in muscle mass. However, some people actually gain body fat. Increased body fat with regular exercise seems counterintuitive, so how does it happen? After vigorous exercise, most people feel justifiably fatigued and hungry. To satiate the post-exercise hunger, it is important to plan for and consume a nutritious meal. Without adequate planning, people often reach for convenience foods such as granola bars, smoothies, candies, or fast foods. Additionally, people may consume a larger amount of food than the body needs because they are very hungry. The end result is that the amount of calories consumed after exercise far exceeds the amount burnt during exercise, thereby leading to increased body fat. I find it helpful to pack a fruit to eat immediately after exercise. This helps calm my hunger until I can find a nutritious meal.

Table 15-2 Calories burned during common exercises

| Exercise[3] | Calories consumed[3] |
|---|---|
| 130 lb. person lifting weights for 1 hour and 30 minutes | 257 |
| 130 lb. person cleaning the house for 2 hours and 35 minutes | 525 |
| 130 lb. persons vacuuming for 1 hour and 30 minutes | 290 |
| 130 lb. person walking leisurely for 1 hour and 20 minutes | 305 |
| 130 lb. person playing tennis for 55 minutes | 380 |
| 130 lb. person washing car for 1 hour and 15 minutes | 220 |
| 130 lb. persons doing aerobic dance for 1 hour and 5 minutes | 430 |
| 160 lb. person working in the garden for 35 minutes | 165 |
| 160 lb. person riding a bike for 1 hour and 25 minutes | 500 |
| 160 lb. person playing golf while walking and carrying clubs for 1 hours | 350 |
| 160 lb. persons doing water aerobics for 1 hour and 15 minutes | 360 |

Table 15-3 Calories in commonly eaten foods

| Food item | Calories[2] |
|---|---|
| 16 oz. mocha coffee with whole milk and mocha syrup | 350 |
| 4 oz. muffin | 500 |
| 2 slices of pepperoni pizza | 850 |
| 3.5 cups of chicken caesar salad | 790 |
| 11 cups of Movie popcorn | 630 |
| 7 oz. slice of cheesecake | 640 |
| 3.5" diameter chocolate chip cookie | 275 |
| 4.5 cups of chicken stir fry | 865 |
| 6" diameter bagel | 350 |
| Cheeseburger | 590 |
| 2 cups of pasta with sauce and 3 large meatballs | 1025 |
| 6.9 oz french fries | 610 |
| 20 oz. soda | 250 |
| Turkey sandwich | 820 |

## Bottom Line on Exercise

- Regular physical exercise has tremendous health benefits.
- Almost all adults should engage in regular physical exercise on most days out of the week.
- Exercise alone is not sufficient to lose weight or maintain a healthy weight.
- A whole-food, plant-based diet is essential to minimize the risk of excess body weight and most chronic diseases.
- Pack a fruit to eat after exercise and then plan for a nutritious meal.

# Chapter 16
# Dining out and Other Helpful Tips to Start Your Plant-Based Journey

Switching from a conventional American diet to a whole-food, plant-based diet can seem overwhelming. After all, we are not just talking about food, but a change in lifestyle. Well-meaning friends and relatives can ease or hinder the transition depending upon their own preferences. Rest assured that adopting a plant-based diet has never been easier. There are now many health-food stores that sell essential ingredients. Many cities have excellent plant-based restaurants. Most ethnic foods are naturally plant-based, and therefore ethnic restaurants are usually a good bet.

In this chapter, I will offer tips and suggestions that will ease your journey into the plant-based world. Once you start eating a whole-food, plant-based diet, you will feel the changes almost immediately. Expect to feel lighter, stronger, and more energized without the heaviness and weighed-down feeling that often follows meals composed of animal products.

Before we start, I would like you to know that I have no financial or other affiliations with any of the products, brands, or restaurants I recommend. I am simply basing my suggestions on what has worked for me and my family.

## Getting Started

Some people ease into plant-based eating over a few weeks, while others make an immediate switch. There is no right or wrong way. It all depends upon your needs and  comfort level. The important thing is to make the switch, whether it is immediate or gradual.

If you are going to make a gradual transition, you can try the following sequence:

- Week 1: Make the switch from refined grains to whole grains as outlined in Chapter 7.
- Week 2: Switch from red meats (beef, lamb, and pork) to plant-based alternative such as tofu, legumes, and vegetables.
- Week 3: Switch poultry products (chicken, eggs, turkey) for plant-based options. Continue to explore recipes using tofu, soy-based products, legumes, and vegetables.
- Week 4: Trade seafood for plant-based options as you continue to try various forms of tofu, legumes, and vegetables.
- Week 5: Switch from dairy to non-dairy milk. (See Transitioning from dairy products)
- Week 6: Switch from dairy to non-dairy yoghurt. (See Transitioning from dairy products)
- Week 7: Switch from dairy cheese to vegan cheese or cheese-free options. (See Transitioning from dairy products)

## Transitioning from Dairy Products

Dairy products are a big part of the western diet as milk, creams, cheese, and yoghurt are frequently used in food preparation. Fortunately, this is one of the easiest transitions to make as there are many wonderful plant-based alternatives.

<u>Milk</u>

There are many types of plant-based milks available: soy, flax, almond, coconut, cashew, hemp. Most of them come in sweetened, unsweetened, plain, and vanilla flavors. Try different types and flavors to see what you like. Avoid sweetened milks as they have added sugar. After trying different milks in different recipes, these are my favorites:

- Coffee & Tea—I love soy milk with my coffee and tea-based drinks as it has the creamiest texture and really enhances the flavor.
- Smoothies—all vegan milks work well.
- Cereal and oatmeal—my family and I really enjoy flax milk as it has a mild and light taste.
- Baking—all vegan milks work well.

<u>Yoghurt</u>

I love eating plain, unsweetened yoghurt and after adopting a plant-based diet, this is the dairy product that I missed the most. I tried the various soy-, almond-, or coconut-based yoghurts commonly sold, but did not care for the taste. They were very sweet with a strong aftertaste. One evening while we were dining with some good friends, they shared with us how much they enjoy their home-made dairy yoghurt. Although it seemed like a daunting and time-consuming task, I decided to try making my own non-dairy yoghurt with soy milk using a yoghurt maker. It turned out to be much easier than I thought, and the taste was fantastic! We sometimes strain the yoghurt to thicken it. My children love it with fresh fruit and agave. It is great in tzatziki, and I also enjoy it plain with spicy Indian food.

Cheese

This one can be tough, as most of the non-dairy cheeses sold in supermarkets leave something to be desired. Having said that, after months of experimentation with various recipes and cookbooks, my family and I have found successful options:

- Grilled cheese: "Chao" vegan cheeses come in various flavors. My kids enjoy these in grilled-cheese sandwiches.
- Pasta: "Chloe's Vegan Italian Kitchen" and "Forks Over knives" cookbooks have several pasta sauces we enjoy. I recommend trying the various sauces in these books to see which ones work for you and your family.
- Pizza: I have not found a good plant-based cheese for pizza. My husband and I order our pizza without cheese and love it! We order thin and crispy pizza crust with tomato sauce, and ask the chef to load it up with our favorite veggies, such as mushrooms, onions, olives, and eggplant. Top it off with arugula and it is excellent!
- Quesadillas or tacos: Quesadillas needs cheese to hold them together. Rather than quesadillas, we now make tacos with veggies and guacamole and they are always a hit! Please see the recipes section.
- Burgers or sandwiches: Rather than using cheese, we use avocados, which provide a similar creamy and flavorful texture.

## Dining Out

There are many excellent plant-based restaurants around the country, and many gourmet chefs and restaurants take great pride in serving healthy plant-based meals. Most restaurants offer some plant-based options and even if there is nothing on the menu, many chefs are happy to put something together. Generally speaking, it is quite easy to find many plant-based options at most ethnic restaurants such as:

- Indian (though the food many contain "ghee", a type of dairy butter)
- Thai, Chinese, Vietnamese, Japanese (though the food may be prepared with fish sauce or beef/chicken broth)
- Greek
- Lebanese
- Spanish
- Italian
- Mexican (though the beans may be prepared with lard)

Even at most restaurant chains such as Subway, Panera, and Chipotle, it is possible to order a nutritious plant-based meal. Gourmet pizzerias are particularly enjoyable as you can simply order your pizza loaded with veggies and skip the cheese. As I mentioned earlier, I love to top mine off with arugula!

Whenever I travel, I love to check out local plant-based restaurants. Here are some of my favorite vegetarian or vegan restaurants around the country.

- Le Pain Quotidien - This Belgian restaurant chain offers many vegan options, which change daily and seasonally.
- Cafe Gratitude in Los Angeles and San Diego. Vegan.
- Mother's in Austin, Texas .Vegetarian and vegan.
- Casa de Luz in Austin, Texas. Vegan and gluten free.
- Vegenation in Las Vegas, Nevada. Vegan.

- Simply Pure in Las Vegas, Nevada. Vegan.
- Wynn and Encore Hotels in Las Vegas. All restaurants at the Wynn and Encore offer gourmet vegan options.
- Sunflower Vegetarian Restaurant in Vienna and Falls Church, Virginia. Vegetarian and vegan.

This list is by no means comprehensive and there are likely many other excellent vegan restaurants around the country. These are just the ones I have had the opportunity to sample so far during my family vacations!

# Chapter 17
# My Family's Favorite Recipes

Before our children were born, my husband and I hardly ever cooked. In fact, we used to avoid cooking as much as we could. Our idea of eating in was ordering take-out food! Over the years, we have started cooking more and more, partly out of concern for our children, and partly to improve our own health. As we have cooked more, we have come to realize how much healthier home-made food can be compared to restaurant or pre-packaged foods. At home, we control how much fat, sugar, and salt we add to the food. Whereas most restaurant and pre-packaged foods are high in all three of these ingredients. As a result, restaurant and pre-packaged foods are much more calorically dense than home-made ones.

Don't feel discouraged if you don't like to cook, don't know how, or don't have the time to cook. Start out gradually and do the best you can. No one can cook every meal, but the more you stick with home-made meals, the better results you will see.

These are some of my family's favorite recipes. They have been thoroughly vetted for their nutritional content (by me), and for taste by my connoisseur husband and children. All of the recipes use whole grains, and minimize the use of added fats and sugar.

## Simple Home-Made Bread

Most commercially-baked breads are made from processed flours rather than whole grains. It is possible to find whole grain breads, however most of these lack freshness and flavor. My husband came up with this bread recipe and it is by far my favorite bread. We make this bread weekly. It is fantastic, especially fresh out of the oven!

### Ingredients

- 4.5 cups white whole wheat flour
- 1 cup rolled oats
- 1/2 cup gluten
- 2 tsp yeast (not instant)
- 1 tbsp salt
- 1/4 cup olive oil
- 1/4 cup sugar
- 1 TBSP lemon juice
- 2.5 cups water

### Preparation

- Mix 2 cups of white whole wheat flour, 1 cup rolled oats, 1/2 cup gluten, and yeast together in a stand mixer.
- Add 2 cups of warm water heated to 110 degrees Fahrenheit. Mix with stand mixer and let the mixture sit for 30 minutes.
- Dough will rise during this time.
- Preheat the oven to 350 degrees.
- After sitting for 30 minutes, add sugar, lemon juice, and olive oil, and mix with stand mixer at low speed.
- Add in 2 cups of white whole flour gradually while mixing. Dough will become harder and pull aways from the sides of the mixing bowl.

- Divide the dough into two halves. Shape it by hand place each into a bread baking dish.
- Turn off the oven which is currently at 350 degrees.
- Place the bread container with dough into the oven and let sit for 30 minutes. No need to cover.
- After dough rises for 30 minutes, set the oven to 350 degrees and bake for 30 minutes
- Remove bread from oven. Remove loaves from baking pan and allow to cool on cooling rack.

## Sweet or Savory Crepes

Do you like crepes? Most commercially-prepared crepes are made from processed flours using eggs and butter. My husband created this healthy recipe in which he uses whole grains without any eggs or butter. This mixture will keep well in the fridge for days. So prepare it ahead of time and make them for breakfast the next day! This is my kids' favorite breakfast!

Ingredients for batter

- 3 cups whole wheat pastry flour
- 1 cup water
- 4-4.5 cups unsweetened plain vegan milk
- 3 teaspoons baking powder
- Mix all ingredients using a hand or stand mixer

Ingredients for filling

- Vegan chocolate chips
- Fresh sliced berries, mangoes, bananas, or peaches

Preparation

- Warm a non stick crepe pan in medium heat. Lightly spray the pan with vegetable oil. Drop a dollop of batter on crepe pan and spread it around to cover the pan. Cook on medium heat for a few minutes. Flip the crepe and cook other side for a few minutes.
- While the second side is cooking, line the middle with about 8-10 vegan chocolate chips until they melt.
- Lay the cooked crepe flat on a plate on top of a plain cloth napkin to absorb excess moisture.
- Add sliced strawberries/bananas or raspberries in the center.
- Roll up the crepe and enjoy!

## Fettuccine with Tomatoes, Cannellini Beans, and Spinach

This is a delicious and satisfying pasta meal. Rather than using creams or meat/fish, we use nutritious tomatoes, legumes, veggies, and pair them with whole grain pasta!

Ingredients

- 3/4 box whole wheat fettuccine
- 3 large beefsteak tomatoes chopped
- 10 peeled crushed garlic cloves
- 3/4 tsp salt
- 1 can chick peas OR cannellini beans OR navy beans (drain and rinse the beans with cold running water)
- 1 medium package of pre-washed baby spinach
- 1 tsp olive oil

Preparation

- Cook pasta al dente according to package instructions.
- Place olive oil in large non-stick pan over medium heat.
- Add garlic, stir frequently, and cook until golden brown (< 1 min).
- Add tomatoes and salt.
- Cover pan with lid and cook on low-med heat until tomatoes become mushy, usually about 15-20 minutes. Stir occasionally.
- Add beans and spinach to pan and cover with lid.
- Once spinach wilts, your sauce is ready.
- Serve the sauce over the pasta and enjoy!

## Quinoa with Black Beans, Corn, & Guacamole

Quinoa is a delicious and nutritious whole grain. It is available in many colors. Some brands require pre-washing while others do not. All types are equally nutritious. In this recipe, I mix quinoa with Mexican seasoning, black beans, and corn and then serve it with guacamole. It always hits the spot!

Ingredients

- 1 cup uncooked quinoa (any color)
- 1 can unsalted black beans, drained and rinsed in fresh water
- 3/4 cup frozen corn
- 1/2 cup chopped red bell peppers
- 1 tsp vegetable oil
- 1/2 tsp salt
- 2 tsp taco seasoning
- 1 tsp lemon or lime juice

Preparation

- Cook quinoa according to package instructions.
- Warm oil in a large non-stick pan on low to medium heat for about 1 minute.
- Add red peppers, seasoning and salt, and stir for about 1-2 minutes.
- Add black beans and corn.
- Cover and simmer on low heat for about 3 minutes until corn is tender
- Add cooked quinoa and mix.
- Add lime/lemon juice according to taste and stir together.
- Serve with a side of home-made guacamole.

## Guacamole

Avocados are nutritious and naturally creamy. Rather than using cheese or heavy creams that are loaded with saturated fats, we make our own guacamole, which is very easy to do. It pairs very well with the taco and quinoa recipes.

<u>Ingredients</u>

- 2 large ripe avocados
- 1/4 tsp finely chopped white onion
- 1/4 tsp granulated garlic (available in the spice section at the local grocery store)
- 1/2 tsp salt
- 1 tbsp chopped cilantro (optional)
- 1 tsp lemon/lime juice

<u>Preparation</u>

- Mash avocados in a bowl.
- Mix in the remaining ingredients and enjoy!

## Black Bean & Mushroom Tacos

My family loves Mexican food. Unfortunately, most of the Mexican food served in restaurants is very oily, cheesy, and salty. Additionally, many restaurants prepare their black or refried beans with lard. Tacos are usually topped with cheese and in this recipe, I substitute cheese with healthier home-made guacamole. This recipe is a hit with everyone and surprisingly easy to make.

<u>Ingredients</u>

- 1 can unsalted black beans, rinsed and strained
- 2 cups chopped shiitake mushrooms (without the stem)
- 2 tsp taco seasoning mix
- ½ tsp salt
- 1/2 tsp vegetable oil
- 1 packet corn tortillas

<u>Preparation</u>

- Warm oil in a medium sized non-stick skillet or wok on medium heat.
- Add mushrooms, taco seasoning mix, and salt.
- Cook mushrooms on medium heat (uncovered) for about 10-15 minutes until tender. Stir every few minutes to prevent burning. The mushrooms will initially release water and once the water has mostly evaporated, they are cooked.
- Add black beans, mix and cook for about 2-3 minutes.
- Warm corn tortillas on a cast iron pan on medium heat for 2 minutes on each side.
- Serve with black bean and mushroom filling and top with guacamole. See guacamole recipe.

## Brown Rice Stir Fry with Veggies and Tofu

I love fried rice but most of the fried rice served in restaurants is very rich in oil and sodium. In this recipe, I minimize the added oil and sodium while enhancing the natural flavor of veggies and spices.

<u>Ingredients</u>

- 1.5 cup uncooked brown rice
- 1 package super firm tofu
- 1 cup frozen peas
- 1 cup frozen corn
- 1/4 cup low sodium soy sauce
- 1/2 tsp Sriracha sauce
- 4 cloves crushed garlic
- 1 tsp crushed ginger
- 1 cups finely chopped pineapple
- 1 tsp olive oil
- 1 cup of chopped cilantro
- 1 cup of chopped scallions

<u>Preparation</u>

- Boil water in a large saucepan. Add rice to boiling water. Cook for about 20-25 minutes until soft. Strain and use for stir fry. Alternatively, you many also use a rice cooker with a brown rice setting.
- Strain tofu and slice in roughly 1 cm cubes.
- Warm a large non-stick skillet and spray with vegetable oil.
- Add sliced tofu and sauté for 5-10 minutes until it is golden brown.
- Warm 2 tsp vegetable oil in large wok on low-medium heat.
- Add garlic and ginger and sauté for about 3 minutes until golden brown.
- Add soy sauce and Sriracha sauce.

- Add all veggies, pineapple and mix together.
- Cover and cook on medium heat for about 10 minutes.
- Mix in rice and tofu.
- Add more soy sauce, Sriracha sauce and lemon juice as desired.
- Garnish with chopped scallions and cilantro.

## Chocolate Chia Seed Pudding

This is a delightful and nutritious pudding that can be enjoyed as a dessert or snack. My children wanted to make it clear that they do not like this recipe (because of chia seeds), but my husband and I love it!

Ingredients

- 1/4 cup cocoa powder
- 8 pitted medjool dates
- 3 cups unsweetened soy, coconut, or almond milk
- 1/3 cup chia seeds
- 1 cup fresh blueberries

Instructions

- Blend cocoa powder, medjool dates, and vegan milk in a high-speed blender such as a Vitamix or Blendtec.
- Add chia seeds and manually mix with a spoon.
- Refrigerate overnight and enjoy!
- I love to eat mine with fresh blueberries.

## Baked Sweet Potato Fries

Kids and adults love French fries with ketchup. However, commercially-cooked fries are deep fried and full of unhealthy fats, salt, and empty calories. Baking retains the nutritious values of potatoes while providing a delicious alternative to frying.

<u>Ingredients</u>

- 2 medium sized baking potatoes or sweet potatoes
- 1 tsp vegetable oil
- 1/2 tsp salt

<u>Preparation</u>

- Wash potatoes thoroughly
- Using a food processor, cut into French fry shapes (Do NOT peel the skin as the skin contains much of the protein and fiber)
- In a large mixing bowl, mix potatoes, salt and oil
- Line a baking tray with parchment paper
- Place potatoes onto baking tray
- Preheat oven to 375 degrees fahrenheit
- Bake for about 30 minutes at 375 degrees until tops are golden brown and crispy
- Serve with ketchup or Sriracha sauce

## Whole Grain Avocado & Tomato Sandwich

This is a very simple and satisfying sandwich that makes for a great snack, lunch, or even breakfast! It is easy to pack and take with you.

Ingredients

- Sliced tomatoes (heirloom tomatoes taste best)
- Sliced avocados
- Whole grain sandwich bread. Most commercially-baked breads are not whole grain. Use the simple bread recipe to make a whole-grain bread.
- Optional: arugula or micro greens.

Preparation

- Use toasted or un-toasted bread according to taste. I like un-toasted bread when it is freshly baked, and toasted otherwise.
- Add a layer of sliced avocados and tomatoes
- Add salt and black pepper to taste
- Optional: top with fresh arugula or micro greens
- Try it as an open or closed sandwich!

## Peanut Butter & Chocolate Chip Cookies

Traditional cookies are very sugary, and buttery and are made with refined flours. This recipe uses whole grains, while minimizing the use of added sugars and fats. My kids gobble these up and I love them with a glass of soy milk or a cup of tea!

Ingredients

- 1 cup whole wheat pastry flour
- 1/2 cup oat flour
- 2 tbsp amaranth flour
- 2 tsp baking powder
- 1 tsp baking soda
- 1/2 tsp salt
- 1/4 cup cane sugar
- 1/2 cup vegan semi-sweet or bittersweet chocolate chips
- 2 tbsp pure maple syrup
- 2 tbsp canola or vegetable oil
- 2/3 cup smooth peanut butter
- 2 tsp pure vanilla extract
- 6 tbsp or 60ml unsweetened vegan milk

Instructions

- Preheat oven to 350
- Using a stand mixer, combine all ingredients
- Use a small cookie scoop to scoop out the dough into 1-2 large baking trays
- Shape the scoops into round cookies
- Bake for 15 minutes until the cookie tops are golden brown
- Allow to cool on a cooling tray
- Enjoy with a cup of soy milk, coffee, or tea

# References

**Introduction**

1.  Health expenditure per Capita. The World Bank website. http://data.worldbank.org/indicator/SH.XPD.PCAP Accessed 9/20/15.
2.  Eat for Health Act Fact sheet. Physicians Committee for Responsible Medicine website. http://pcrm.org/sites/default/files/pdfs/Eat-for-Health-Factsheet-7-16.pdf Accessed September 19, 2015.

**Chapter 1. What Is a Healthy Weight and Why Does It Matter?**

1.  Obesity and overweight. World Health Organization website. http://www.who.int/mediacentre/factsheets/fs311/en/ Updated January 2015. Accessed 9/25/15.
2.  Obesity and overweight. Centers for Disease Control and Prevention website. http://www.cdc.gov/nchs/fastats/obesity-overweight.htm Last reviewed January 21, 2014. Updated September 30, 2015. Accessed 9/25/15.

3.  Diabetes latest. Centers for Disease Control and Prevention website. http://www.cdc.gov/features/diabetesfactsheet/ Reviewed June 17, 2014. Updated June 17, 2014. Accessed 10/6/15.

4.  Heart Disease. Centers for Disease Control and Prevention website. http://www.cdc.gov/heartdisease/facts.htm Reviewed August 10, 2015. Updated August 10, 2015. Accessed 9/24/15.

5.  About heart disease and stroke. Health and Human Services website.http://millionhearts.hhs.gov/abouthds/cost-consequences.html Accessed September 30, 2015.

6.  Esselstyn CB Jr. Is the Present Therapy for Coronary Artery Disease the Radical Mastectomy of the Twenty-First Century? *The Am J Cardiol.* 2010;106: 902-904.

7.  Bray GA. Obesity in adults: Health hazards. In: UpToDate, Post TW (Ed), UpToDate, Waltham, MA. (Accessed on September 19, 2015.)

8.  Bray GA. Determining body fat composition in adults. In: UpToDate, Post TW (Ed), UpToDate, Waltham, MA. (Accessed on September 20, 2015.)

9.  Bray GA. Obesity in adults: Prevalence, screening and evaluation. In: UpToDate, Post TW (Ed), UpToDate, Waltham, MA. (Accessed on September 19, 2015.)

10. Rolfes S, Pinna K, Whitney E. Energy Balance and Body Composition. In: *Understanding normal and clinical nutrition.* 9th ed. Belmond, CA: Wadsworth; 2012:241-259.

## Chapter 2. Overview of the Health Benefits of a Plant-Based Diet

1.  Meat Free Diets Best for Weight loss.Physicians Committee for Responsible Medicine website. http://www.pcrm.org/health/medNews/meat-free-weight-loss-diet July 13, 2015. Accessed on October 5, 2015.

2.  Campbell T, Campbell II T. (2006-06-01). *The China Study: The Most Comprehensive Study of Nutrition Ever Conducted and the Startling Implications for Diet, Weight Loss and Long-Term Health.* BenBella Books, Inc.. Kindle Edition.

3.  Vegetarian Diets Increase Metabolism. Physicians Committee for Responsible Medicine website. http://www.pcrm.org/health/

medNews/vegetarian-diets-increase-metabolism July 30, 2015. Accessed on October 5, 2015.

4.  Rolfes S, Pinna K, Whitney E. Table of Food Composition. In: *Understanding normal and clinical nutrition*. 9th ed. Belmond, CA: Wadsworth; 2012:H1-H87

5.  McCulloch DK. Clinical presentation and diagnosis of diabetes mellitus in adults. In: UpToDate, Post TW (Ed), UpToDate, Waltham, MA. (Accessed on October 6, 2015.)

6.  Levitsky L, Misra M. Epidemiology, presentation, and diagnosis of type 1 diabetes mellitus in children and adolescents. In: UpToDate, Post TW (Ed), UpToDate, Waltham, MA. (Accessed on October 9, 2015.)

7.  Pietropaolo P. Pathogenesis of Type 1 diabetes mellitus. In: UpToDate, Post TW (Ed), UpToDate, Waltham, MA. (Accessed on October 6, 2015.)

8.  McCulloch DK, Pietropaolo P. Prevention of type 1 diabetes mellitus. In: UpToDate, Post TW (Ed), UpToDate, Waltham, MA. (Accessed on October 6, 2015.)

9.  Diabetes latest. Centers for Disease Control and Prevention website. http://www.cdc.gov/features/diabetesfactsheet/ Reviewed June 17, 2014. Updated June 17, 2014. Accessed 10/6/15.

10. Laffel L, Svoren B. Epidemiology, presentation, and diagnosis of type 2 diabetes mellitus in children and adolescents In: UpToDate, Post TW (Ed), UpToDate, Waltham, MA. (Accessed on October 7, 2015.)

11. Barnard ND, Cohen J, Jenkins DJ, et al. A low-fat vegan diet improves glycemic control and cardiovascular risk factors in a randomized clinical trial in individuals with type 2 diabetes. Diabetes Care 2006;29:1777-83.

12. Lee YM, Kim SA, Lee IK, Kim JG, Park KG, et al. (2016) Effect of a Brown Rice Based Vegan Diet and Conventional Diabetic Diet on Glycemic Control of Patients with Type 2 Diabetes: A 12-Week Randomized Clinical Trial. PLoS ONE 11(6): e0155918. doi:10.1371/journal.pone.0155918

13. Satija A, Bhupathiraju SN, Rimm EB, Spiegelman D, Chiuve SE, Borgi L, et al. (2016) Plant-Based Dietary Patterns and Incidence of Type 2 Diabetes in US Men and Women: Results from Three Prospective Cohort Studies. PLoS Med 13(6): e1002039. doi: 10.1371/journal.pmed.1002039

14. Kaplan NM, Mount DB. Potassium and hypertension. In: UpToDate, Post TW (Ed), UpToDate, Waltham, MA. (Accessed on October 28, 2015.)

15. Meat consumption and cancer risk. Physicians Committee for Responsible Medicine website. http://www.pcrm.org/health/cancer-resources/diet-cancer/facts/meat-consumption-and-cancer-risk Accessed on October 7, 2015.

16. Chen, WY. Factors that modify breast cancer risk in women. In: UpToDate, Post TW (Ed), UpToDate, Waltham, MA. (Accessed on October 7, 2015.)

17. Virus Found in Dairy Linked to Breast Cancer. Physicians Committee for Responsible Medicine website. http://www.pcrm.org/health/medNews/virus-in-dairy-linked-to-breast-cancer September 17, 2015. Accessed October 7, 2015.

18. Fat Linked to Breast Cancer Risk. Physicians Committee for Responsible Medicine website. http://www.pcrm.org/health/medNews/fat-linked-to-breast-cancer-risk June 13, 2014. Accessed October 7, 2015.

19. IARC Monographs evaluate consumption of red meat and processed meat. International Agency for Research on Cancer website. http://www.iarc.fr/en/media-centre/pr/2015/pdfs/pr240_E.pdf Published October 26, 2015. Accessed October 26, 2015.

20. Meat Eater's Guide: Report. Meat and your health. Environmental Working Group website. http://www.ewg.org/meateatersguide/a-meat-eaters-guide-to-climate-change-health-what-you-eat-matters/meat-and-your-health/ Accessed October 27, 2015.

21. Q&A on the carcinogenicity of the consumption of red meat and processed meat. International Agency for Research on Cancer website. http://www.iarc.fr/en/media-centre/iarcnews/pdf/Monographs-Q&A_Vol114.pdf Accessed October 26, 2015.

22. Sartor AO. Risk factors for prostate cancer. In: UpToDate, Post TW (Ed), UpToDate, Waltham, MA. (Accessed on October 7, 2015.)

23. Milk and Prostate Cancer: The Evidence Mounts. Physicians Committee for Responsible Medicine website. http://www.pcrm.org/health/health-topics//milk-and-prostate-cancer-the-evidence-mounts (Accessed on October 8, 2015.)

24. Olek MJ, Mowry E. Pathogenesis and epidemiology of multiple sclerosis. In: UpToDate, Post TW (Ed), UpToDate, Waltham, MA. (Accessed on October 9, 2015.)

25. Rosen HN. Calcium and vitamin D supplementation in osteoporosis. In: UpToDate, Post TW (Ed), UpToDate, Waltham, MA. (Accessed on October 13, 2015.)

26. Bolland MJ, Leung W, Tai V et al. Calcium intake and risk of fracture: systematic review. *BMJ*. 2015;351:h4580.

27. Tai V, Leung W, Grey A, et al. Calcium intake and bone mineral density: systematic review and meta-analysis. *BMJ*. 2015;351:h4183.

28. Michaëlsson K. Calcium supplements do not prevent fractures. *BMJ*. 2015;351:h4825.

## Chapter 3. Prominent Research Studies Supporting Whole-Food, Plant-Based Diets

1. Campbell T, Campbell II T. (2006-06-01). *The China Study: The Most Comprehensive Study of Nutrition Ever Conducted and the Startling Implications for Diet, Weight Loss and Long-Term Health*. BenBella Books, Inc.. Kindle Edition.

2. Ornish DM, Brown SE, Scherwitz LW, et al. Can lifestyle changes reverse coronary heart disease? The Lifestyle Heart Trial. *Lancet*. 1990;336:129-33.

3. Ornish DM, Scherwitz LW, Billings JH, et al. Intensive Lifestyle changes for reversal of coronary heart disease. *JAMA*. 1998;280:2001-2007.

4. Esselstyn CB Jr. Updating a 12-year experience with arrest and reversal therapy for coronary heart disease (an overdue requiem for palliative cardiology). Am J Cardiol. 1999;84:339-341,A8.

5. Esselstyn CB Jr. Resolving the Coronary Artery Disease Epidemic through Plant-Based Nutrition. *Prev Cardiol*. 2001;4:171-177.

6. Esselstyn CB Jr, Gendy G, Doyle J, et al. A way to reverse CAD? *J Family Pract*. 2014;63:356-164.

7. Esselstyn CB Jr. In Cholesterol Lowering, Moderation Kills. *Cleve Clinic J of Med*. 2000;67(8): 560-564

8. Esselstyn CB Jr. Is the Present Therapy for Coronary Artery Disease the Radical Mastectomy of the Twenty-First Century? *The Am J Cardiol*. 2010;106: 902-904.

9.  Tonstad S, Butler T, Yan R, Fraser GE. Type of vegetarian diet, body weight and prevalence of type 2 diabetes. *Diabetes Care.* 2009;32(5):791-796.

## Chapter 4. Impact of Eating Animal-based Foods on Our Environment and Fellow Animals

1.  Boseley, S. Processed meats rank alongside smoking as cancer causes – WHO. *The Guardian.* October 26, 2015. http://www.theguardian.com/society/2015/oct/26/bacon-ham-sausages-processed-meats-cancer-risk-smoking-says-who?CMP=fb_gu Accessed on October 27, 2015.
2.  Health & Environmental Implications of U.S. Meat Consumption & Production. Johns Hopkins Bloomer School of Public Health website. http://www.jhsph.edu/research/centers-and-institutes/johns-hopkins-center-for-a-livable-future/projects/meatless_monday/resources/meat_consumption.html Accessed October 20, 2015.
3.  Meat Eater's Guide: Report. Other Meat Concerns: Antibiotics, Hormones and Toxins. Environmental Working Group website. http://www.ewg.org/meateatersguide/a-meat-eaters-guide-to-climate-change-health-what-you-eat-matters/other-meat-concerns-antibiotics-hormones-and-toxins/ Accessed October 27, 2015.
4.  Walsh, B. The Triple Whopper Environmental Impact of Global Meat Production. *Time.* December 16, 2013 http://science.time.com/2013/12/16/the-triple-whopper-environmental-impact-of-global-meat-production/ Accessed October 26, 2015.
5.  Meat Eater's Guide: Report. Climate and Environmental Impacts. Environmental Working Group website. http://www.ewg.org/meateatersguide/a-meat-eaters-guide-to-climate-change-health-what-you-eat-matters/climate-and-environmental-impacts/ Accessed October 26, 2015.
6.  Scheer R, Moss D. How Does Meat in the Diet Take an Environmental Toll? *Scientific American.* Dec 28, 2011. http://www.scientificamerican.com/article/meat-and-environment/ Accessed Oct 20, 2011.

7. Meat Eater's Guide: Report. What you eat matters. Environmental Working Group website. http://www.ewg.org/meateatersguide/a-meat-eaters-guide-to-climate-change-health-what-you-eat-matters/ Accessed October 26, 2015.

## Chapter 5. What about Other Diets Such as Mediterranean, Low-Carb, Paleo, and Okinawan?

1. M Nestle. Mediterranean diets: historical and research overview. Am J Clin Nutr. 1995 Jun;61(6 Suppl):1313S-1320S.
2. A Keys. Mediterranean diet and public health: personal reflections. Am J Clin Nutr. 1995 Jun;61(6 Suppl):1321S-1323S.
3. G E Voukiklaris, A Kafatos, A S Dontas. Changing prevalence of coronary heart disease risk factors and cardiovascular diseases in men of a rural area of Crete from 1960 to 1991. Angiology. 1996 Jan;47(1):43-9.
4. High Blood Pressure Facts. Centers for Disease Control and Prevention website.http://www.cdc.gov/bloodpressure/facts.htm Last reviewed February 19, 2015. Updated February 19, 2015. Accessed 4/9/16.
5. Campbell T, Campbell II T. (2006-06-01). *The China Study: The Most Comprehensive Study of Nutrition Ever Conducted and the Startling Implications for Diet, Weight Loss and Long-Term Health*. BenBella Books, Inc.. Kindle Edition.
6. Mozaffarian D, Benjamin EJ, Go AS, Arnett DK, Blaha MJ, Cushman M, de Ferranti S, Després J-P, Fullerton HJ, Howard VJ, Huffman MD, Judd SE, Kissela BM, Lackland DT, Lichtman JH, Lisabeth LD, Liu S, Mackey RH, Matchar DB, McGuire DK, Mohler ER 3rd, Moy CS, Muntner P, Mussolino ME, Nasir K, Neumar RW, Nichol G, Palaniappan L, Pandey DK, Reeves MJ, Rodriguez CJ, Sorlie PD, Stein J, Towfighi A, Turan TN, Virani SS, Willey JZ, Woo D, Yeh RW, Turner MB; on behalf of the American Heart Association Statistics Committee and Stroke Statistics Subcommittee. Heart disease and stroke statistics—2015 update: a report from the American Heart Association [published online ahead of print December 17, 2014]. Circulation. doi: 10.1161/CIR.0000000000000152.

7.  M de Lorgeril, S Renaud, N Mamelle, P Salen, J L Martin, I Monjaud, J Guidollet, P Touboul, J Delaye. Mediterranean alpha-linolenic acid-rich diet in secondary prevention of coronary heart disease. Lancet. 1994 Jun 11;343(8911):1454-9.

8.  M de Lorgeril, P Salen, J L Martin, I Monjaud, J Delaye, N Mamelle. Mediterranean diet, traditional risk factors, and the rate of cardiovascular complications after myocardial infarction: final report of the Lyon Diet Heart Study. Circulation. 1999 Feb 16;99(6):779-85.

9.  Esselstyn CB Jr, Gendy G, Doyle J, et al. A way to reverse CAD? *J Family Pract.* 2014;63:356-164.

10. R Estruch, E Ros, J Salas=Salvado, M I Covas, D Coreela, F Aros, E Gomez-Gracia, V Ruiz-Gutierrez,M Fiol, J Lapetra, R M Lamuela-Raventos, L Serra-Majem, X Pinto, J Basora, M A Munoz, J V Sorli, J A Martinez, M A Martinez-Gonzalez, PREMIDED Study Investigators. Primary prevention of cardiovascular disease with a Mediterranean diet. N Engl J Med. 2013 Apr 4;368(14):1279-90.

11. Supplement to: Estruch R, Ros E, Salas-Salvadó J, et al. Primary prevention of cardiovascular disease with a Mediterranean diet. N Engl J Med 2013;368:1279-90. DOI: 10.1056/ NEJMoa1200303

12. B J Willcox, D C Willcox, H Todoriki, A Fujiyoshi, K Yano, Q He, J D Curb, M Suzuki. Caloric restriction, the traditional Okinawan diet, and healthy aging: the diet of the world's longest-lived people and its potential impact on morbidity and life span. Ann N Y Acad Sci. 2007 Oct;1114:434-55.

13. Joyce, C. Japanese get a taste for Western food and fall victim to obesity and early death. *The Telegraph.* September 4, 2006. http:// www.telegraph.co.uk/news/health/news/3342882/Japanese-get-a-taste-for-Western-food-and-fall-victim-to-obesity-and-early-death.html Accessed on April 8, 2016.

14. D. Craig Willcox PhD, Bradley J. Willcox MD, Hidemi Todoriki PhD & Makoto Suzuki MD, PhD (2009) The Okinawan Diet: Health Implications of a Low-Calorie, Nutrient-Dense, Antioxidant-Rich Dietary Pattern Low in Glycemic Load, Journal of the American College of Nutrition, 28:sup4, 500S-516S, DOI: 10.1080/07315724.2009.10718117

15. N S Gavrilova, L A Gavrilov. Comments on Dietary Restriction, Okinawa Diet and Longevity. Gerontology. 2012 Apr; 58(3): 221–223.

16. Teresa T. Fung, ScD; Rob M. van Dam, PhD; Susan E. Hankinson, ScD; Meir Stampfer, MD, DrPH; Walter C. Willett, MD, DrPH; and Frank B. Hu, MD, PhD Low-Carbohydrate Diets and All-Cause and Cause-Specific Mortality: Two Cohort Studies. *Ann Intern Med.* 2010;153(5):289-298

17. Noto H, Goto A, Tsujimoto T, Noda M. Low-Carbohydrate Diets and All-Cause Mortality: A Systematic Review and Meta-Analysis of Observational Studies. Manzoli L, ed. *PLoS ONE.* 2013;8(1):e55030. doi:10.1371/journal.pone.0055030.

18. Jordi Merino, Richard Kones, Raimon Ferré, Núria Plana, Josefa Girona, Gemma Aragonés, Daiana Ibarretxe, Mercedes Heras and Luis Masana (2013). Negative effect of a low-carbohydrate, high-protein, high-fat diet on small peripheral artery reactivity in patients with increased cardiovascular risk. British Journal of Nutrition, 109, pp 1241-1247. doi:10.1017/S0007114512003091.

19. Barnett TD, Barnard ND, Radak TL. Development of symptomatic cardiovascular disease after self-reported adherence to the Atkins diet. J Am Diet Assoc. 2009 Jul;109(7):1263-5.

20. M M Smith, E T Trexler, A J Sommer, B E Starkoff, S T Devor. Unrestricted Paleolithic Diet is Associated with Unfavorable Changes to Blood Lipids in Healthy Subjects. International Journal of Exercise Science 7(2) : 128-139, 2014.

## Chapter 6. Commonly Cited Barriers to Plant-Based Eating

1. New Vegan Celebrities of 2013. Physicians Committee for Responsible Medicine website. http://www.pcrm.org/health/diets/ffl/employee/newly-vegan-celebrities-of-2013 (Accessed on October 4, 2015.)

2. Darby, L. The Real-Life Diet of a Vegan NFL Defensive Lineman. *GQ.* http://www.gq.com/story/vegan-diet-of-nfl-player-david-carter August 11, 2015. Accessed October 4, 2015.

3. Karni, A. Bill Clinton's vegan Las Vegas adventure. Politico website. http://www.politico.com/story/2016/02/bill-clinton-las-vegas-meals-219484 Accessed February 21, 2016.

4. A brief history of tobacco. CNN website. http://edition.cnn.com/US/9705/tobacco/history/ Accessed October 4, 2015.

5. Sharkey, J. What Flying Was Like Before the Smoke Cleared. *The New York Times*. February 23, 2015. http://www.nytimes.com/2015/02/24/business/what-airlines-were-like-before-the-smoke-cleared.html? r=0 Accessed October 4, 2015.

6. Fee E, Brown TM. Hospital Smoking Bans and Their Impact. *Am J Public Health*. 2004; 94(2): 185

7. Esselstyn CB Jr. Resolving the Coronary Artery Disease Epidemic through Plant-Based Nutrition. *Prev Cardiol*. 2001;4:171-177.

8. Government Support for Unhealthful Foods. Physicians Committee for Responsible Medicine website. http://www.pcrm.org/health/reports/agriculture-and-health-policies-unhealthful-foods Accessed October 6, 2015.

9. Agricultural Policies Versus Health Policies. Physicians Committee for Responsible Medicine website. http://www.pcrm.org/health/reports/agriculture-and-health-policies-ag-versus-health Accessed October 6, 2015.

10. Eat for Health Act Fact sheet. Physicians Committee for Responsible Medicine website. http://pcrm.org/sites/default/files/pdfs/Eat-for-Health-Factsheet-7-16.pdf Accessed September 19, 2015.

## Chapter 7. Brief Nutrition Outline

1. Rolfes S, Pinna K, Whitney E. Energy Balance and Body Composition. In: *Understanding normal and clinical nutrition*. 9th ed. Belmond, CA: Wadsworth; 2012:241-259.

## Chapter 8. Carbohydrates - Friend or Foe?

1. Rolfes S, Pinna K, Whitney E. The Carbohydrates: Sugars, Starches, and Fibers. In: Understanding normal and clinical nutrition. 9th ed. Belmond, CA: Wadsworth; 2012:97-121.

2. Moss, M. *Salt Sugar Fat: How the Food Giants Hooked Us*. New York: Random House; 2013.

3. Rolfes S, Pinna K, Whitney E. Energy Balance and Body Composition. In: *Understanding normal and clinical nutrition*. 9th ed. Belmond, CA: Wadsworth; 2012:241-259.

4. What is a Whole Grain? Whole Grains Council website. wholegrainscouncil.org/whole-grains-101/what-is-a-whole-grain Accessed October 20, 2015.

5.  Rolfes S, Pinna K, Whitney E. Planning a healthy diet. In: Understanding normal and clinical nutrition. 9th ed. Belmond, CA: Wadsworth; 2012:50-51.

6.  Nutrients in Wheat Flour: Whole, Refined and Enriched. Whole Grains Council website. http://wholegrainscouncil.org/files/backup_migrate/WGvsEnriched2011.pdf Accessed on October 20, 2015.

7.  Nutrients in Rice: Whole, Refined and Enriched. Whole Grains Council website. http://wholegrainscouncil.org/files/RiceWGvsEnriched2011.pdf Accessed on October 20, 2015.

8.  Whole grain Fact Sheet. European Food Information council website. http://www.eufic.org/article/en/expid/whole-grain-fact-sheet/ Accessed October 20, 2015.

9.  Whole Grains A to Z. Whole Grains Council website. http://wholegrainscouncil.org/whole-grains-101/whole-grains-a-to-z Accessed October 20, 2015.

10.  Oats – January Grain of the Month. Whole Grains Council website. http://wholegrainscouncil.org/whole-grains-101/oats-january-grain-of-the-month Accessed October 20, 2015.

11.  Wheat July Grain of the Month. Whole Grains Council website. http://wholegrainscouncil.org/whole-grains-101/wheat-july-grain-of-the-month Accessed October 20, 2015.

12.  Whole White Wheat FAQ. Whole Grains Council website. http://wholegrainscouncil.org/whole-grains-101/whole-white-wheat-faq Accessed October 29, 2015.

13.  Schuppan D, Dieterich W. Pathogenesis, epidemiology, and clinical manifestations of celiac disease in adults. In: UpToDate, Post TW (Ed), UpToDate, Waltham, MA. (Accessed on October 21, 2015.)

14.  Kelly C. Diagnosis of celiac disease in adults. In: UpToDate, Post TW (Ed), UpToDate, Waltham, MA. (Accessed on October 21, 2015.)

15.  Ciclitira PJ. Management of celiac disease in adults. In: UpToDate, Post TW (Ed), UpToDate, Waltham, MA. (Accessed on October 21, 2015.)

16.  Gluten Free Whole Grains. Whole Grains Council website. http://wholegrainscouncil.org/whole-grains-101/gluten-free-whole-grains Accessed on October 21, 2015.

# Chapter 9. Fat and Cholesterol

1. Moss, Michael (2013-02-26). Salt Sugar Fat: How the Food Giants Hooked Us (Kindle Locations 2951-2955). Random House Publishing Group. Kindle Edition.
2. Rolfes S, Pinna K, Whitney E. The Lipids: Triglycerides, Phospholipids, and Sterols. In: Understanding normal and clinical nutrition. 9th ed. Belmond, CA: Wadsworth; 2012:133-203.
3. Rosenson R. Measurement of blood lipids and lipoproteins. In: UpToDate, Post TW (Ed), UpToDate, Waltham, MA. (Accessed on November 25, 2015.)
4. Castelli WP. Making practical sense of clinical trial data in decreasing cardiovascular risk. *Am J Cardiol.* 2001;88(4A): 16F-20F
5. Pignone M. Treatment of lipids (including hypercholesterolemia) in primary prevention. In: UpToDate, Post TW (Ed), UpToDate, Waltham, MA. (Accessed on November 17, 2015.)
6. Rosenson R. Treatment of lipids (including hypercholesterolemia) in secondary prevention. In: UpToDate, Post TW (Ed), UpToDate, Waltham, MA. (Accessed on November 17, 2015.)
7. Rind D, Hayward R. Intensity of lipid lowering therapy in secondary prevention of cardiovascular disease. In: UpToDate, Post TW (Ed), UpToDate, Waltham, MA. (Accessed on November 17, 2015.)
8. Framingham Heart Study website. https://www.framinghamheartstudy.org Accessed November 17, 2015.
9. Go AS, Mozaffarian D, Roger VL, Benjamin EJ, Berry JD, Borden WB, Bravata DM, Dai S, Ford ES, Fox CS, Franco S, Fullerton HJ, Gillespie C, Hailpern SM, Heit JA, Howard VJ, Huffman MD, Kissela BM, Kittner SJ, Lackland DT, Lichtman JH, Lisabeth LD, Magid D, Marcus GM, Marelli A, Matchar DB, McGuire DK, Mohler ER, Moy CS, Mussoli- no ME, Nichol G, Paynter NP, Schreiner PJ, Sorlie PD, Stein J, Turan TN, Virani SS, Wong ND, Woo D, Turner MB; on behalf of the American Heart Association Statistics Committee and Stroke Statistics Subcommittee. Heart disease and stroke statistics—2013 update: a report from the American Heart Association.Circulation. 2013;127:e6-e245.

10. Gillman M. Dietary Fat. In: UpToDate, Post TW (Ed), UpToDate, Waltham, MA. (Accessed on November 15, 2015.)

11. Press D, Alexander M. Prevention of dementia. In: UpToDate, Post TW (Ed), UpToDate, Waltham, MA. (Accessed on November 15, 2015.)

12. Saturated Fat. Physicians Committee for Responsible Medicine website. http://www.pcrm.org/health/saturated-fat Accessed on November 15, 2015.

13. The FDA takes step to remove artificial trans fats in processed foods. U.S. Food and Drug Administration website. http://www.fda.gov/NewsEvents/Newsroom/PressAnnouncements/ucm451237.htm Published June 16, 2015. Accessed on November 15, 2015.

14. Campbell T, Campbell II T. (2006-06-01). *The China Study: The Most Comprehensive Study of Nutrition Ever Conducted and the Startling Implications for Diet, Weight Loss and Long-Term Health.* BenBella Books, Inc.. Kindle Edition.

15. Ornish DM, Brown SE, Scherwitz LW, et al. Can lifestyle changes reverse coronary heart disease? The Lifestyle Heart Trial. *Lancet.* 1990;336:129-33.

16. Ornish DM, Scherwitz LW, Billings JH, et al. Intensive Lifestyle changes for reversal of coronary heart disease. *JAMA.* 1998;280:2001-2007.

17. Esselstyn CB Jr. Updating a 12-year experience with arrest and re- versal therapy for coronary heart disease (an overdue requiem for palliative cardiology). Am J Cardiol. 1999;84:339-341,A8.

18. Esselstyn CB Jr. Resolving the Coronary Artery Disease Epidemic through Plant-Based Nutrition. *Prev Cardiol.* 2001;4:171-177.

19. Esselstyn CB Jr, Gendy G, Doyle J, et al. A way to reverse CAD? *J Family Pract.* 2014;63:356-164.

20. Trends in Intake of Energy and Macronutrients in Adults From 1999-2000 Through 2007-2008. Centers for Disease Control and Prevention website. http://www.cdc.gov/nchs/data/databriefs/db49.htm November 2010. Accessed on November 16, 2015.

21. U.S. Department of Health and Human Services and U.S. Department of Agriculture. 2015 – 2020 Dietary Guidelines for Americans. 8th Edition. December 2015. Available at http://health.gov/dietaryguidelines/2015/guidelines/.

22. IARC Monographs evaluate consumption of red meat and processed meat. International Agency for Research on Cancer

website. http://www.iarc.fr/en/media-centre/pr/2015/pdfs/
pr240_E.pdf Published October 26, 2015. Accessed October 26,
2015.

23. Q&A on the carcinogenicity of the consumption of red meat
and processed meat. International Agency for Research on
Cancer website. http://www.iarc.fr/en/media-centre/iarcnews/
pdf/Monographs-Q&A_Vol114.pdf      Accessed October 26,
2015.

24. Meat consumption and cancer risk. Physicians Committee for
Responsible Medicine website. http://www.pcrm.org/health/
cancer-resources/diet-cancer/facts/meat-consumption-and-
cancer-risk Accessed on October 7, 2015.

## Chapter 10. Why Protein Is Not Always the Answer

1. Rolfes S, Pinna K, Whitney E. Protein: Amino Acids. In:
Understanding normal and clinical nutrition. 9th ed. Belmond,
CA: Wadsworth; 2012:173-202.

2. The Protein Myth. Physicians Committee for Responsible
Medicine website. http://www.pcrm.org/health/diets/vegdiets/
how-can-i-get-enough-protein-the-protein-myth Accessed on
November 10, 2015.

3. U.S. Department of Agriculture, Agricultural Research Service.
2014. Nutrient Intakes from Food and Beverages: Mean
Amounts Consumed per Individual, by Gender and Age, What
We Eat in America, NHANES 2011-2012.

4. Questions and Answers on Dietary Supplements. U.S. Food and
Drug Administration website. http://www.fda.gov/Food/
DietarySupplements/QADietarySupplements/
default.htm#FDA_role   Last updated April 28, 2015. Accessed
on November 11, 2015.

## Chapter 11. What about All Those Vitamins & Minerals?

1. Questions and Answers on Dietary Supplements. U.S. Food and
Drug Administration website. http://www.fda.gov/Food/
DietarySupplements/QADietarySupplements/
default.htm#FDA_role   Last updated April 28, 2015. Accessed
on November 11, 2015.

2.  Fairfield K. Vitamin supplementation in disease prevention. In: UpToDate, Post TW (Ed), UpToDate, Waltham, MA. (Accessed on November 29, 2015.)

3.  Hochberg L, Stone J. Folic acid supplementation in pregnancy. In: UpToDate, Post TW (Ed), UpToDate, Waltham, MA. (Accessed on November 29, 2015.)

4.  Folate Dietary Supplement Fact Sheet. National Institutes of Health website. Reviewed December 14, 2012. https://ods.od.nih.gov/factsheets/Folate-HealthProfessional/#h4 Accessed December 2, 2015.

5.  Vitamin D Fact Sheet for Health Professionals. National Institutes of Health website. https://ods.od.nih.gov/factsheets/VitaminD-HealthProfessional/#h3 Reviewed November 10, 2014. Accessed November 30, 2015.

6.  Dawson-Hughes B. Vitamin D deficiency in adults: Definition, clinical manifestations, and treatment. In: UpToDate, Post TW (Ed), UpToDate, Waltham, MA. (Accessed on November 30, 2015.)

7.  Campbell, T. Colin; Thomas M. Campbell II (2006-06-01). The China Study: The Most Comprehensive Study of Nutrition Ever Conducted and the Startling Implications for Diet, Weight Loss and Long-Term Health (p. 232). BenBella Books, Inc.. Kindle Edition.

8.  Vitamin B12 Dietary Supplement Fact Sheet. National Institutes of Health website. https://ods.od.nih.gov/factsheets/VitaminB12-HealthProfessional/#h3 Reviewed June 24, 2011. Accessed on December 2, 2015.

9.  Don't Vegetarians Have Trouble Getting Enough Vitamin B12? Physicians Committee for Responsible Medicine website. http://www.pcrm.org/health/diets/vegdiets/dont-vegetarians-have-trouble-getting-enough Accessed on December 2, 2015.

10. Calcium Dietary Supplement Fact Sheet. National Institutes of Health website. https://ods.od.nih.gov/factsheets/Calcium-HealthProfessional/#h7 Reviewed November 21, 2013. Accessed on December 2, 2015.

11. Calcium in Plant-Based diets. Physicians Committee for Responsible Medicine website. http://www.pcrm.org/health/diets/vsk/vegetarian-starter-kit-calcium Accessed on December 2, 2015.

12. Lewiecki E. Prevention of Osteoporosis. In: UpToDate, Post TW (Ed), UpToDate, Waltham, MA. (Accessed on December 2, 2015.)

13. Bolland MJ, Leung W, Tai V et al. Calcium intake and risk of fracture: systematic review. *BMJ*. 2015;351:h4580.

14. Tai V, Leung W, Grey A, et al. Calcium intake and bone mineral density: systematic review and meta-analysis. *BMJ*. 2015;351:h4183.

15. Michaëlsson K. Calcium supplements do not prevent fractures. *BMJ*. 2015;351:h4825.

16. Pazirandeh S,Burns DL, Griffin IJ. Overview of dietary trace minerals. In: UpToDate, Post TW (Ed), UpToDate, Waltham, MA. (Accessed on December 2, 2015.)

17. Wolin KY, Colditz GA. Cancer Prevention. In: UpToDate, Post TW (Ed), UpToDate, Waltham, MA. (Accessed on December 2, 2015.)

18. Sodium:q&a. Centers for Disease Control and Prevention website. http://www.cdc.gov/salt/pdfs/Sodium_QandA.pdf Published 02/2014. Accessed on December 5, 2015.

19. Institute of Medicine (US) Committee on Strategies to Reduce Sodium Intake; Henney JE, Taylor CL, Boon CS, editors. Strategies to Reduce Sodium Intake in the United States. Washington (DC): National Academies Press (US); 2010. 4, Preservation and Physical Property Roles of Sodium in Foods. Available from: http://www.ncbi.nlm.nih.gov/books/NBK50952/

20. Sodium and Food Sources. Centers for Disease Control and Prevention website. http://www.cdc.gov/salt/food.htm Last updated August 21, 2014. Accessed on December 5, 2015.

21. CDC Vital signs. Centers for Disease Control and Prevention website. http://www.cdc.gov/VitalSigns/pdf/2012-02-vitalsigns.pdf Published February 7, 2012. Accessed on December 5, 2015.

22. Sodium: the facts. Centers for Disease Control and Prevention website. http://www.cdc.gov/salt/pdfs/Sodium_Fact_Sheet.pdf Original publication date: 06/2010. Updated: 02/2013. Accessed on December 5, 2015.

23. Kaplan NM. Salt intake, salt restriction, and primary (essential) hypertension. In: UpToDate, Post TW (Ed), UpToDate, Waltham, MA. (Accessed on December 4, 2015.)

24. Vitamin C Fact Sheet for Health Professionals. National Institutes of Health website. https://ods.od.nih.gov/factsheets/VitaminC-HealthProfessional/ Reviewed June 5, 2013. Accessed on December 7, 2015.

25. Sexton DJ, McClain MT. The common cold in adults: Treatment and prevention. In: UpToDate, Post TW (Ed), UpToDate, Waltham, MA. (Accessed on December 7, 2015.)

## Chapter 12. Healthy Eating Habits and Our Food Environment

1. Weight loss: Gain control of emotional eating. Mayo Clinic website. http://www.mayoclinic.org/healthy-lifestyle/weight-loss/in-depth/weight-loss/art-20047342 October 03, 2015. Accessed on December 9, 2011.

2. Portion Distortion. National Institutes of Health website. https://www.nhlbi.nih.gov/health/educational/wecan/eat-right/portion-distortion.htm Last Updated: April 1, 2015. Accessed December 10, 2015.

3. Young LR. *the portion teller smart size your way to permanent weight loss.* New York: Morgan Road Books; 2005.

4. World Famous Fries. McDonald's website. http://www.mcdonalds.com/us/en/food/product_nutrition.snackssides.6050.small-french-fries.html Accessed December 10, 2015.

5. Quarter Pounder with Cheese. McDonald's website. http://www.mcdonalds.com/us/en/food/product_nutrition.burgerssandwiches.7.quarter-pounder-with-cheese.html Accessed December 10, 2015.

6. Double Quarter Pounder with Cheese. McDonald's website. http://www.mcdonalds.com/us/en/food/product_nutrition.burgerssandwiches.3426.double-quarter-pounder-with-cheese.html Accessed December 10, 2015.

7. Your McDonald's Meal's BFF. McDonald's website. http://www.mcdonalds.com/us/en/food/product_nutrition.beverages.520.cocacola-classic-small.html Accessed December 10, 2015.

8. Pizza Hut Nutritional Guide. Pizza Hut website. http://www.pizzahut.com/assets/w/nutrition/BrandStandardNutritionalInformationFINAL111314.pdf Accessed December 10, 2015.

9. Wansink, B. *Slim by Design: Mindless Eating Solutions for Everyday Life.* New York: HarperCollins; 2014.

10. Arumugam, N. How Size And Color Of Plates And Tablecloths Trick Us Into Eating Too Much. *Forbes.* http://www.forbes.com/sites/nadiaarumugam/2012/01/26/how-size-and-color-of-plates-and-tablecloths-trick-us-into-eating-too-much/ Published January 26, 2012. Accessed December 11, 2015.

## Chapter 13. Dessert - How Sweet Is Too Sweet?

1. Heart Health Benefits of Chocolate. Cleveland Clinic website. http://my.clevelandclinic.org/services/heart/prevention/nutrition/food-choices/benefits-of-chocolate Reviewed 01/12. Accessed December 14, 2015.

## Chapter 14. Beware of Liquid Calories

1. Coca-cola website. Accessed January 4, 2016.
2. Starbucks website. Accessed January 5, 2016.
3. Rolfes S, Pinna K, Whitney E. Table H-1 Table of Food Composition. In: *Understanding normal and clinical nutrition.* 9th ed. Belmond, CA: Wadsworth; 2012:H1-H87.

## Chapter 15. Why Exercise Alone Is Not Enough

1. Peterson, DM. The benefits and risks of exercise. In: UpToDate, Post TW (Ed), UpToDate, Waltham, MA. (Accessed on January 4, 2016.)
2. U.S. Department of Health and Human Services and U.S. Department of Agriculture. 2015 – 2020 Dietary Guidelines for Americans. 8th Edition. December 2015. Available at http://health.gov/dietaryguidelines/2015/guidelines/.
3. Portion Distortion. National Institutes of Health website. https://www.nhlbi.nih.gov/health/educational/wecan/eat-right/portion-distortion.htm Last Updated: April 1, 2015. Accessed January 4, 2016.

# Index

Made in the USA
Lexington, KY
31 October 2016